Tap Tap and Grind

Secrets your dentist wants you to know

By Dr. Samuel Schlesinger DDS

Copyright © 2021

All Rights Reserved

Edited by Kristin Pierri

Dedicated to my niece Maddie and my nephew Jake

Preface

"Why didn't anyone tell me this before?"

This question used to excite me. It provided me with an opportunity to educate my patients and help them gain control of their oral health. At the same time, it allowed me to demonstrate my understanding of dentistry. However, as time went on, my excitement turned into concern. Why were so many people not aware of basic oral health and at the very least, their own oral health? Was it their previous dental experience? Was it passed on from their parents? Was it financially driven? Was it insurance driven? Was it quickly glossed over in school or at the family doctor's office? Like most things, especially in dentistry, it was all of the above. This is why I decided to write this book. I was tired of hearing this question from my patients. I did a quick search on the internet and realized there were no books out there to help people understand what was going on in their mouth. I have tried to cram in as much knowledge as I could in the simplest way possible so that after reading this book, everything at the dentist will finally make sense.

My treatment philosophy is simple. I want every patient to be able to blow out their birthday candles without their teeth falling out at 100 years old. Name me something that you use as frequently as your mouth and teeth. Every time you smile, frown, laugh, talk or eat, you use your mouth and teeth. Perhaps the most important of these is the smile. It's the first thing you notice on a person and is the symbol that is rated with the highest positive emotional content. I want my patients to be happy and to love their smile. So, how do we get there? The first step is overall health. This includes regular visits to both your family doctor and to your dentist. As we age, our capacity to heal diminishes and we can no longer keep up with the wear and tear that our body experiences. This extends to our mouth and teeth as well. That's where we come in! First we take care of your fundamental needs with cleanings and getting rid of any decay. Next, comes the fun part! If you are unhappy with your smile, we can help restore your self-confidence and happiness with Invisalign, implants, crowns or veneers to deliver the smile of your dreams.

Writing this book allows me to reach more people because I can only see so many patients in a day. With so much information available at our fingertips these days and with the myriad of health-conscious trends, I believe there is not enough emphasis placed on the importance of oral health as part of overall health. Now is the time to gain control of your oral health. 2021 is the year when we all finally start flossing.

Table of Contents

1. Medical, Dental and Social History 1
2. New Patient Exam / Complete Oral Exam 2
3. X-rays 4
4. Children's Teeth 9
    - The first 2 years 9
    - Baby bottle tooth decay 10
    - Tooth Eruption 11
    - Trauma 12
5. Fluoride (taken from ADA, 5) 14
6. Oral Hygiene 16
    - Flossing 16
    - Mouthwash 17
    - Brushing 18
7. Cleanings and Gum Disease 19
8. How long will this last? 22
9. Cavities 24
10. Crowns and Veneers 29
11. Whitening 34
12. Gum Recession 39
    - Abrasions 40
    - Abfractions 41
    - Erosion 42
13. Nightguards 44

14. Invisalign/Orthodontics 48

15. Extractions 51

- Wisdom teeth 52

16. Root Canals 54

17. Implants 58

18. Pregnancy 66

19. Medications 69

- Painkillers 69

- Antibiotics 72

- Antibiotic premedication 73

- Other common medications 74

20. Post-op Instructions 76

- Oral Surgery 76

- Implants 77

- Sedation (with Triazolam) 78

- Nightguards 81

- Invisalign 82

21. References 84

Medical, Dental and Social History

"Why are you asking me all these questions? I'm just getting a cleaning."

Just like going to your family doctor's office, we need a thorough medical history from you. This involves a complete list of health conditions, a full medication list (including supplements) and any known or potential allergies. It may not seem important at the dental office but trust me, it is. Your medical history gives us insight into your dental health and may impact the management of dental issues. We use many different tools, materials, medications and anaesthetics during your treatment which can cause undue stress to your body and can potentially interact with certain health conditions or medications you may be taking. Before we can deliver any dental treatment, we need to ensure you are safe while you are in our care. Our first priority is always your safety. We ask because we care.

We will also take your blood pressure and vitals. Believe it or not, most cases of hypertension are first seen at the dentist. This is because people will have routine cleanings at their dental office more frequently than visiting their family doctor for an annual physical.

Many dental procedures can cause bleeding (teeth cleaning, gum treatment, extractions or fillings involving the gum area) which can introduce bacteria that is present in the mouth into the bloodstream. For most people, this is not a problem. However, for some people, this can have serious consequences unless precautions are taken. We will discuss antibiotic premedication in more detail in the chapter on common medications.

It is also important for us to gather information about your dental history. This will include details about any recent dental treatment, past dental complications and oral hygiene routines.

Lastly, we will review your social history. This includes information about your diet, occupational stressors, tobacco use and alcohol use. Your social history allows us to put dental problems in context so we can approach your care effectively and holistically. Remember, the body is all connected. Your oral health impacts your general health and your general health impacts your oral health.

New Patient Exam / Complete Oral Exam

Why are we so quick to go to our family doctor when something looks or feels unusual on our bodies other than in our mouth? Is it because we don't bother to look? No! It is because we don't know what we're looking for!

The new patient exam or complete oral exam is by far the most important appointment a patient can have at the dentist. This is both done at your first visit to a new dental office as well as periodically at your current office depending on the frequency that your dentist sets for you. The common frequency for a new complete exam varies from 2 to 5 years. This is not the same as a cleaning check-up where the dentist pops in for a few minutes. Those check-ups are to review any new x-rays and address any acute issues or significant changes that we see since your last visit. We only have 5 minutes or less to do these checks due to everyone's schedule. Sometimes we may see many changes that cannot be addressed in the limited time we have and we recommend that you come back for either a complete exam or more time to discuss what is going on. Cleaning check-ups can be anywhere from 3 to 12-month intervals and the frequency is unique to the patient and is set by your dentist.

As part of the complete oral exam or new patient exam, x-rays are taken (or sometimes x-rays are transferred over from a previous office if they were recent enough) as well as intraoral photos using a digital camera. Sometimes an intraoral scan is taken as well. We take intraoral pictures of your mouth so you can see what we see. We take you on a tour of your mouth which is important because it familiarizes you with what is normal and what is not. We want as much information as possible to ensure nothing is missed. With all this information, we will have the benefit at the next complete exam to compare not only x-rays but pictures as well to see what has changed and the speed that things are changing. This is where recession, wear, nightguards, crowding etc. can be evaluated and compared. We can even measure this digitally by comparing previous intraoral scans.

New Patient Exam / Complete Oral Exam

I give my patients as much time as they need for these appointments and I often get in trouble from my front desk for it. I never rush this appointment. It is an opportunity for both doctor and patient to get to know and understand each other. This is the time to explain, ask questions and address your concerns. At the end of this appointment, we go through what work needs to be done, what can be done and possibilities in the future. Ultimately the decision of what you do and the speed at which you do it is yours. What is of greatest importance is that you leave informed of what is going on in your mouth.

X-rays

"I don't want x-rays today. I'll do them next time."

While many dental professionals might brush this off to avoid confrontation and a potential argument, I see it as an opportunity to educate. I have seen countless patients who fall into a "no x-rays" label. They go years in the same office without taking x-rays because clinicians become burnt out from asking and the patient also becomes burnt out from being asked. We need to address this early before it becomes a habit. Some patients will sign a form that says they rejected x-rays today and are aware of the risks and consequences. Unfortunately, you cannot sign off on neglect. It is not right to continue to treat someone who refuses x-rays for longer than is appropriate and by doing so, dental professionals are enabling that behaviour. So please listen to your health care provider when it comes to x-ray frequency - *we take them for you, not for us.*

In order to maintain and evaluate your oral health, we need regular x-rays so that we can see what our eyes cannot. The whole point of going to the dentist is to catch things early so they don't become a bigger, more invasive and more expensive issue. We cannot see through teeth, gums or bone yet - we are still working on the technology to do so. Until that day comes, we have to rely on x-rays. The frequency of x-rays is determined by your dentist and is specific to you.

So, what type of x-rays are taken and why? There are five types of dental x-rays typically taken to evaluate your dental health, depending on what we are trying to see.

Periapical x-rays

Periapical x-rays show the whole tooth, from the crown (chewing surface) to beyond the root (below the gum line). These are taken for any areas of concern that we see like signs of infection, potential need for a root canal, to assess bone structures and during orthodontic/ Invisalign treatment to ensure there is no root shortening occurring due to teeth moving too quickly. Periapical x-rays are also taken of your upper and lower front teeth every 3 to 5 years.

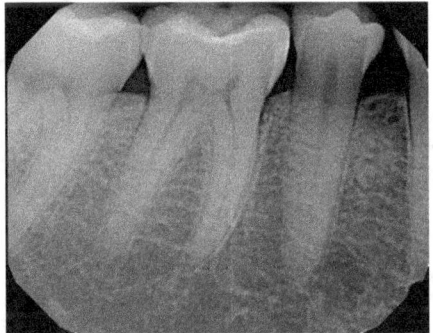

Figure 1: Periapical x-ray

Bitewing x-rays (aka cavity checking x-rays)

Bitewing x-rays capture the crown as well as half of their roots and supporting bone. They are used to detect decay, bone loss and calculus build up. Bitewings are taken every 1 to 3 years depending on your history.

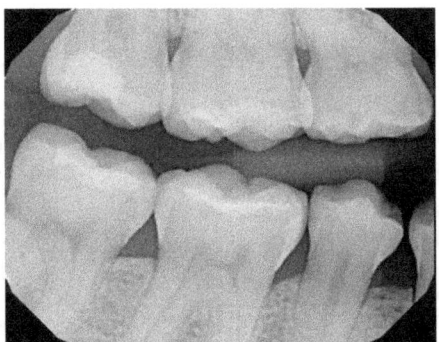

Figure 2: Bitewing x-ray

Cephalometric x-ray

A cephalometric x-ray captures an image of the side of the skull. It is commonly used for orthodontics to evaluate the need for movement in different teeth and their relation with the jaw and skull.

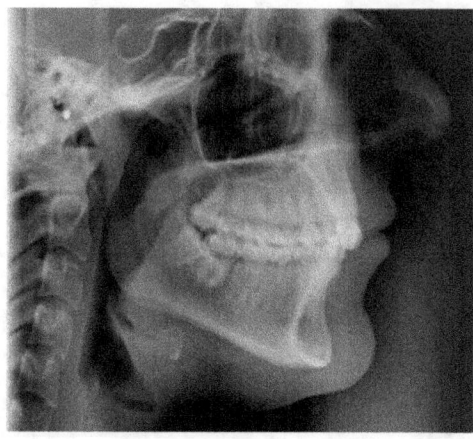

Figure 3: Cephalometric x-ray

Panoramic x-ray

A panoramic x-ray gives us a broad anatomical overview and history of your mouth. It also shows us your jaw joints, nerves and sinuses. It is commonly used for early detection of oral cancer, diseases of the jaw bone, gum disease, tooth and jaw development, impacted wisdom teeth and sinus problems.

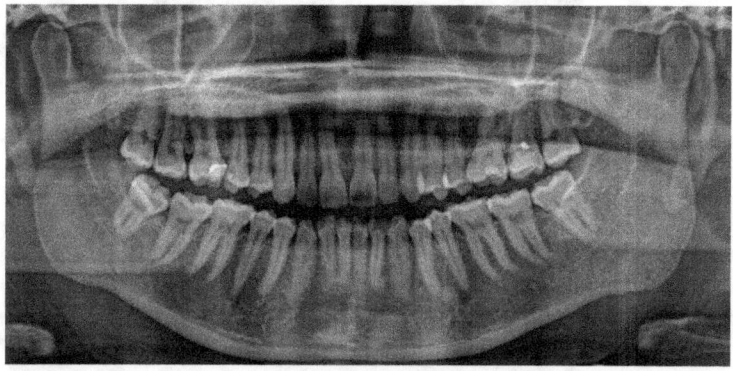

Figure 4: Panoramic x-ray

Oftentimes, we may see something on this x-ray that will lead us to take a periapical because we want a more detailed view of a specific tooth to assess for potential infection. Panoramic x-rays are taken every 3 to 5 years.

Cone Beam CT Scan (or CBCT)

A CBCT is a 3D x-ray. It is only done on an as needed basis for anything that cannot be diagnosed with the 2D x-rays listed above. It provides 3D information about how close a nerve is for an extraction, potential fractures, infections, root canal teeth and large surgeries involving implants. This is different than a medical grade CT. Figure 5 shows a wisdom tooth that is impacted horizontally – it allows us to visualize how close the nerve is before going ahead with surgery. X-rays are also taken during certain dental procedures and as part of follow-ups for treatment. Some examples include:

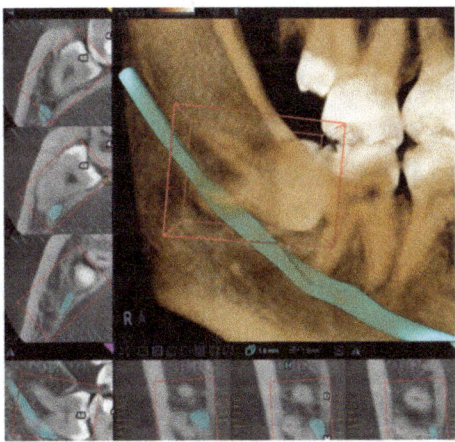

Figure 5: CBCT scan of lower right Wisdom Tooth

- during a root canal to measure the length of the roots, verify all nerves are found and to troubleshoot
- during implant placement to check depth, angulation and proximity to any important anatomy
- during crown/veneer inserts to verify proper seating either before or after they are cemented
- follow ups for root canals to ensure timely healing
- follow ups for implants to ensure stability and to catch any significant changes throughout the first few years of chewing

- follow ups for Invisalign treatment to ensure there is no root shortening occurring due to teeth moving too quickly

Lastly, any trauma needs to be followed up with x-rays to evaluate for any changes in the nerve that may lead to a root canal. There may be other reasons that your dentist decides to take a diagnostic x-ray but they are always in your best interest if it is recommended.

And now, the question that is on everyone's mind: are x-rays safe? Of course they are!

First you need to make the distinction between a medical x-ray and a dental x-ray. Dental x-rays use a fraction of the radiation that medical grade x-rays do. Digital x-rays use even lower amounts with an almost 90% reduction in exposure compared to traditional film x-rays. Getting your average cavity checking x-rays is equivalent to the same radiation that you get in daily life from the sun, your cell phone and other sources. To put it in perspective, an airplane ride from Toronto to London to go visit the Queen will expose you to the same radiation as 16 dental x-rays and that is not counting the airport security scanner which can be as much as 1000 times what is used for a medical chest x-ray. Simply put, dental x-rays are safe and are for your benefit so please take them when they are needed! (Taken from Kois, 1)

You might be wondering - if x-rays are so safe, why do we have to wear a lead apron and why does the hygienist or assistant run out of the room to hide behind the wall? First, we have you wear the lead apron for your safety to limit scatter radiation from the x-ray (which is minimal) because we want to be extra careful to ensure there's no radiation exposure to sensitive parts of the body like your thyroid gland. And why don't we stay in the room? We take many x-rays throughout the day so for safety we try not to expose ourselves more than we have to. But sometimes we do for kids to get a proper x-ray but we will also wear a lead apron in the room at the same time. We want to make sure it is safe for both patients and staff.

Children's Teeth

When do I take my child to the dentist for the first time? When should they start brushing? When should they start flossing? Is this normal? Shouldn't my child have more teeth at this age? Should I use toothpaste?

There are so many questions when it comes to children's teeth that I could devote an entire book to this topic alone. However, that is not the goal here. The goal is to give you as much information in the simplest way possible so you have the tools to not only empower yourself but also to pass that on to your children.

Let's start at the beginning. Birth! When babies are born, the first thing you should know about are natal and neonatal teeth. Natal teeth are present at birth and should be removed because they will interfere with breast feeding and are usually supernumerary (extra) teeth. You can remove these at the hospital or at your dental office. Neonatal teeth can erupt in the first 30 days after birth and should also be removed with your dentist if they are deemed as extra teeth.

The first 2 years

So when should I bring my baby in to see the dentist? You should bring your baby in as soon as that first tooth erupts, so 6 to 12 months. The goal of the first few visits is twofold – it is to get your child comfortable with a new environment and to answer any questions you may have about their dental care. Going to the dentist for the first time can be scary for anyone so those first few appointments are very important to create a positive experience and association.

When should I start brushing my baby's teeth? As soon as that first tooth erupts! No toothpaste, just some water on a baby brush or finger brush after meals and before bedtime. Again, the key here is to get your baby accustomed to oral hygiene and brushing. Even before getting that first tooth, you should use a damp gauze/cloth or finger brush to wipe your baby's gums to get them used to the experience. The key is to never force brushing on your child so they don't form a negative association with it. You want it to be a positive experience. There are lots of books, songs, videos, toys that can help in this regard. Be firm but not forceful. You don't need to use toothpaste until after the age of 2. Start with a small rice grain sized amount of fluoridated toothpaste (high risk of decay) or non-fluoridated (low risk) and gradually upgrade to a pea sized amount around age 3 or when they can successfully spit. If your child initially swallows some of the toothpaste, do not worry. Such small amounts won't have any harmful effect. Always supervise brushing to minimize the amount of toothpaste that gets swallowed.

As teeth begin to come in (teething), your baby may experience symptoms that can make you think something is wrong. A rise in temperature, drooling, diarrhea, loss of appetite and a rash are all common. These symptoms come and go pretty quickly. Obviously if these symptoms persist or get worse, visit your paediatrician to rule out anything else. Chilled teething rings can make your child more comfortable during teething.

Baby bottle tooth decay

If there is one thing that I cannot stress enough, do not let your child fall asleep with a bottle containing milk, water with honey or a sugary drink. This also applies to falling asleep while breastfeeding.

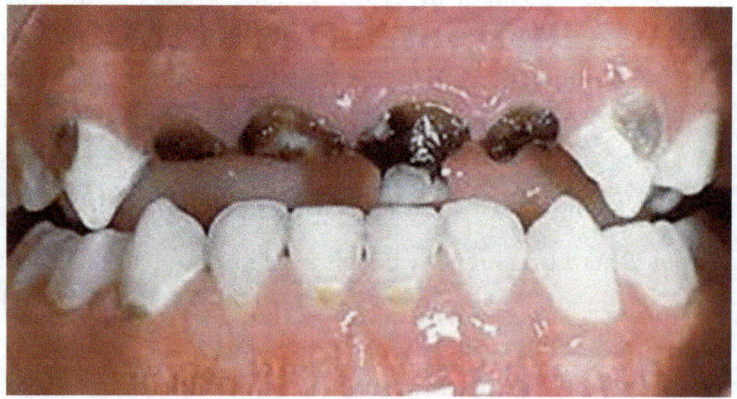

Figure 6: baby bottle syndrome Tooth Decay

I know as parents sleep is very scarce and you will do anything to get some sleep but please avoid doing this.

There can be serious repercussions. Make sure your baby drinks from a cup when they are able to, avoid breastfeeding before bed after the first tooth erupts and brush after having anything sugary. The type of cavities that arise from this are very aggressive (as seen in Figure 6 – taken from the ADA – Patient Smart - 2), hard to treat and are often referred to a specialist.

Losing baby teeth prematurely can lead to speech problems, poor eating habits, crooked teeth and damaged adult teeth. Baby teeth are very important because they hold the place for adult teeth and are crucial in the development of a child's bite.

Tooth Eruption

So when do baby teeth come out? And is this normal?

Figure 7 and 8 outlines typical tooth eruption times. Keep in mind that these are ranges and can be different for each person (Taken from the ADA – Mouthhealthy, 3)

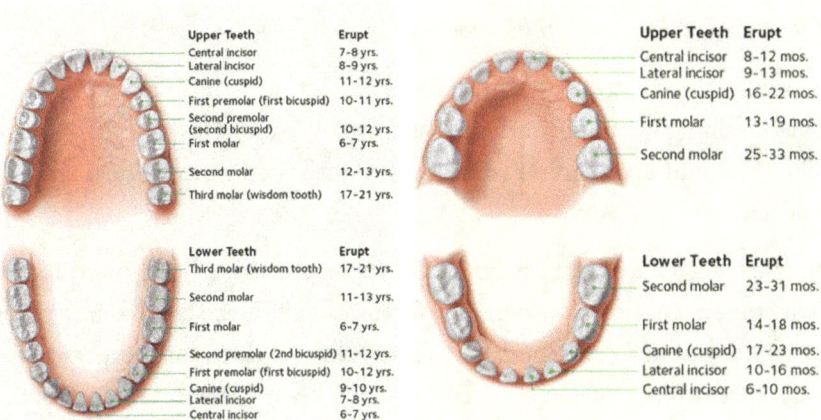

Figure 7: Baby teeth eruption times   *Figure 8: Permanent teeth eruption times*

Just like other developmental trends, girls tend to get teeth faster than boys. Generally lower teeth come in before upper teeth of the same kind.

With kids, be on the lookout for adult teeth coming in before the baby teeth they are replacing fall out. This happens most commonly with the lower adult central incisors and they'll usually come in towards the tongue, as seen in Figure 9 (Taken from HuffPost, 4).

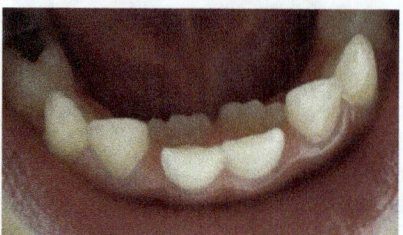

Figure 9: Over-retained baby teeth

This is an indication to remove the baby teeth so that the adult teeth can come back into position otherwise they will develop into the wrong spot. You can give it a week or two to see if the teeth fall out naturally, if not then you should go see your dentist to have them removed. Please do not attempt to remove the teeth yourself - you can break the tooth or even worse, damage the adult tooth coming in.

Trauma

"Oh no, my kid fell and broke a tooth. What do I do?"

Let's talk briefly about trauma. Let's face it, kids are clumsy. They're always falling, tripping and getting into trouble. Broken teeth, teeth falling out and lip lacerations are what dentists commonly deal with for children.

So, your kid fell and cut his lip and chipped a tooth - how do you know what you should do and when you should do it? First, see how bad the lip laceration is. Small cuts heal by themselves but deep cuts and cuts that involve the border of the lips may require stitches. Make sure your child's tetanus shots are up-to-date. Damage to teeth can sometimes be obvious and sometimes they will need the opinion of a dentist to determine what is going on. Small chips at the edges of teeth do not require immediate attention. However once those chips become large, extend below gums, expose a nerve, cause a lot of pain or interfere with the bite then you need to see the dentist sooner rather than later.

If a baby tooth falls out, there is no rush because we never put baby teeth back in. However, if an adult tooth falls out then you have to act quickly. Pick it up by the crown (try not to touch the root part to avoid disturbing any live tissue), place it in milk or back into the tooth socket and go straight to the dentist. The key number to remember is 60 minutes. If you can get that tooth back into the socket in less than 60 minutes, it has the best chance of survival and turning out normally. Beyond this, the tooth will need a root canal. The longer the elapsed time beyond 60 minutes, the less chance of success we'll have of putting the tooth back in the mouth.

Fluoride (taken from ADA, 5)

As a kid, you may remember having the dreaded fluoride rinse at the end of your cleanings. Just like holding a plank, those were probably the longest 60 seconds of your life. But did you ever wonder why you had to do it? No one ever told me, I just did as I was told.

So, what exactly is fluoride? Fluoride is a naturally occurring mineral in nature that is found in all water sources. It tends to be more concentrated in oceans compared to lakes or rivers. But why do we use it in dentistry? We use it because it can help prevent tooth decay. It also protects your teeth in different ways:

- It makes your teeth more resistant to acid attack from bacteria.
- It prevents bacteria from sticking to your teeth.
- It makes it harder for bacteria to survive.
- It promotes tooth building (remineralization).
- It prevents tooth destruction (demineralization).

The US Health and Human Services department in 2015 recommended 0.7mg/L (or 0.7 parts per million) of fluoride as the perfect balance between reducing tooth decay and minimizing potential dental fluorosis. Dental fluorosis is a change in the physical appearance of teeth due to regular ingestion of fluoride, from any source, when teeth are developing under the gums (typically the first 8 years of life). It is most commonly seen as small white spots on teeth. Fluorosis does not affect the health of teeth – it's just cosmetic.

Most communities have been fluoridating their water for years, however there are some communities that have changed their policies in the last few years and what we are seeing is a significant increase in tooth decay in those regions. Check with your local community to confirm whether your water is fluoridated or not.

What if I use a water filter system? The most common filter is a Brita filter. Brita filters or any carbon-based filters only remove trace amounts of fluoride so you still get the benefit. Other systems like under the sink filtration may remove more and you have to check depending on the system. If you mainly drink bottled water, you may not be getting enough fluoride as well. Most bottled water has no fluoride but check the labelling to be sure.

The fluoride in toothpaste and mouth rinse is usually sodium fluoride, sodium monofluoro-phosphate or stannous fluoride. Look out for these when looking for supplementing your fluoride. If you recall, the recommended level of fluoride in drinking water is 0.7ppm but that is for fluoride that is ingested. Over-the-counter toothpaste commonly has 1000-1500 ppm, prescription toothpaste can have 5000ppm, daily mouth rinses containing 0.05% sodium fluoride will have 230ppm (recommended as a daily rinse for high cavity risk individuals over 6 years old) and professional varnishes and gels can have upwards of 22,600ppm. These are all not ingested and just help coat the surfaces of the teeth, more extrinsic rather than intrinsic.

Typically, dentists will recommend an in-office fluoride rinse, gel or varnish at least once a year for children under 18 and for adults who are prone to tooth decay. For certain health conditions, custom fluoride trays for home use may also be recommended.

Oral Hygiene

"Should I brush first or should I floss first?"

This is one of the most common questions that I get asked. A recent study published in the Journal of Periodontology (2018, 6) suggests that flossing first may be more beneficial. Although there is no consensus as yet within the dental community, I would recommend flossing before brushing. The logic is you are removing and bringing anything stuck in between the teeth to the surface so you can brush everything away.

Let's take a step back now and review the basics of good oral hygiene, in the order that they should occur.

Flossing

No matter how well you brush, your toothbrush cannot reach the tight spaces between your teeth and under the gum line. This is why flossing is so important.

Some important things to keep in mind when flossing:

- Don't be frugal. You need about 18 inches to floss properly. You want a clean bit of floss for each tooth. Why? If you use just one bit of floss over and over again, you can spread bacteria and food particles in one part of your mouth to other parts where it may not have been.

- Be gentle. Aggressive flossing can harm your gums. Use a rubbing motion to guide the floss gently between your teeth. When the floss reaches the gum line, curve the floss against the tooth to make a c-shape.

If you just can't get into the habit of flossing, consider using another type of interdental cleaner such as a proxybrush, a wooden wedge plaque remover or a water flosser. Consult with your dentist or hygienist to find out what is best for you.

Mouthwash

Is mouthwash really necessary? For most people, mouthwash is not considered a necessary part of their oral health routine and it is definitely not a substitute for brushing and flossing. No matter what a mouthwash claims it can do, only brushing and flossing can remove plaque from your teeth. However, there is no harm in using a mouthwash a few times a week. For some people (those prone to cavities or gum disease and those with certain medical conditions), mouthwash may be a necessary part of their daily routine. Always check with your dentist to see what is recommended for you.

When it comes to mouthwash, there are some key points to remember:

- Choose a mouthwash that is alcohol free. Alcohol destroys bad (and good) bacteria in the mouth and can dry out your mouth. It can also reduce your saliva production.

- Never give mouthwash to children younger than 6 years of age – they may end up inadvertently swallowing more than they spit out.

- If you have open sores or oral lesions in your mouth, do not use mouthwash. Consult with your dentist first.

- Mouthwash only masks bad breath - it does not deal with the underlying causes of bad breath. If you suffer from chronic bad breath, check with your dentist to find a long term solution.

It is natural to think of mouthwash as the last step of your routine, after brushing and flossing. However, the better way is to use mouthwash before brushing. Since toothpaste has a higher concentration of fluoride than mouthwash, you want that to remain on your teeth as long as possible. Rinsing with mouthwash after brushing can "wash" about the valuable fluoride left behind from brushing.

Brushing

Brushing should be the last step in your oral hygiene routine.

When it comes to brushing your teeth, there are some basic principles to bear in mind.

- Brush your teeth twice a day, morning and night. Don't rush - it takes about 2 minutes to get the job done right. Brush all surfaces of a tooth – outside, inside and biting surfaces.

- Don't brush right after eating. Wait 30 minutes before brushing, especially if you have had something acidic.

- Don't forget your tongue. Your tongue harbours bacteria, which can contribute to bad breath. Brush your tongue daily with a toothbrush or tongue scraper.

- Use a soft-bristled toothbrush or electric toothbrush. Brushing too hard with hard bristles can harm your gums. And yes, size does matters – choose a toothbrush that fits your mouth and hand comfortably.

- After brushing, always rinse your toothbrush with water and allow to air dry in an upright position. If you cover a wet toothbrush, it can promote the growth of bacteria, mold and yeast.

- Replace your toothbrush every 3 months, or sooner if the bristles flay or become irregular. If you get sick, always replace your toothbrush when you are better.

When it comes to brushing, technique matters. How you brush your teeth can make a big difference. Review your brushing technique with your dentist or hygienist to ensure you are doing it properly.

Recent studies indicate that you should not rinse after brushing. Instead, simply spit out any remaining toothpaste. Sounds weird, right? The rationale is that rinsing after brushing will wash away the protective fluoride that has adhered to your teeth. Ideally, you should not eat, drink or rinse for 30 minutes after brushing your teeth.

Cleanings and Gum Disease

Why do I need a cleaning in the first place? How often do I need to get a cleaning? Why do my gums bleed? Why do I need to floss? Why are you poking my gums? What do those numbers mean?

These are just some of the common questions we get when it comes to regular cleanings. Some people love cleanings, some hate them and some don't care. One thing is certain though, we all need regular cleanings. Even with all the tools and aids we can use at home, we cannot clean every area of our mouth properly. We are in a constant battle with bacteria when it comes to our mouth. Plaque (the soft clear film of bacteria that sits on top of your teeth) can be removed with flossing and brushing at home but once it hardens to create tartar (concrete-like substance), you need to have it professionally removed at the dental office. It only takes about 48 short hours for plaque to become tartar. Tartar build up can put your teeth and gums in jeopardy for dental disease. Regular dental cleanings give us an opportunity to catch things early before they become something more serious. It is always preferable (less invasive and less expensive) to be preventative as opposed to reactionary when it comes to dental disease.

Cleaning frequencies can vary from 3 to 12 month intervals. Your dental professional will decide which category you fall in. If you are high risk and have a complicated medical and dental history, you will need to be seen more often than if you've never had a filling before and are otherwise healthy. Dental cleanings are usually done by a hygienist. The hygienist will begin by reviewing your medical history and doing a physical exam of your mouth using a small mirror. Next, they will remove any plaque and tartar around your gum line using a scaler (scraping tool). You will hear scraping but this is normal. The more tartar build up you have, the more they will have to scrape. The hygienist will also floss your teeth to determine if there are any trouble areas where gums may bleed. Finally, the hygienist will use a gritty toothpaste to remove any surface stains. You may also get a fluoride treatment during your cleaning. X-rays, gum measurements, intra-oral pictures and a check up with the dentist may also be done at this visit. While many patients have dental insurance, it is imperative to remember that we are treating you, not your insurance. Your insurance may only cover one cleaning a year but you may need two or three cleanings a year to maintain your oral health. Insurance is just a subsidy to help you out.

Part of determining your frequency of cleanings has to do with gum measurements and gum disease. If gum disease exists, it's important to know if it is gingivitis (only affects the gums) or periodontitis (affects both gums and bone). Things may start off as gingivitis but if they are not addressed, it can progress to periodontitis. Gingivitis treatment is as simple as regular cleanings and practicing regular oral hygiene at home. Periodontitis treatment can be more complicated depending on the severity and can involve multiple cleaning appointments with freezing, medication and even surgery. Your risk of developing periodontitis can involve a lot of different factors like systemic diseases, genetics, medications, recreational drugs, bruxism and socioeconomic status. Everyone is different and will require a personalized oral health maintenance plan.

Gum measurements are commonly done to determine the health of your gums and see if there are any areas you are having trouble maintaining. This is done by placing a dental probe beside your tooth beneath your gumline to measure the pocket depth of the groove between your gums and teeth. We generally take these measurements annually but it can be sooner depending on your oral health and treatment. In a healthy mouth, the golden number is between 1 and 3 millimeters (mm) because this is what you can maintain at home with proper brushing, flossing and rinsing. Measurements of 4mm indicate that the tissue is inflamed and that some dental treatment may be necessary. Numbers greater than 5mm indicate that intervention is required to prevent disease. Once pockets get deeper (beyond 5mm), only we can clean those areas properly. Even so, we are limited as to how far we can reach. We can only successfully get to 5-6mm pockets with our instruments. Beyond this, surgical intervention is usually required to access the areas of bacteria and infection. We use these measurements to help determine your cleaning frequency - if your pockets are all 3mm then you don't have to come in as often as someone with 5mm pockets everywhere.

Now that you understand what happens at a dental cleaning and why, I hope that you will feel more comfortable at your next visit – who knows, you might even look forward to it! Lastly, don't be afraid of asking your hygienist or dentist any questions you might have. There is no such thing as a stupid question when it comes to your oral health. This is your time.

How long will this last?

"This will last forever, right? If I do this once, then I'll never have to do it again?"

There is nothing we do in your mouth that you cannot undo. Read that sentence again. Nothing lasts forever. If what we are replacing (your natural tooth) didn't last forever then why would the next best thing last forever or longer? If your natural tooth did not last your entire life then why would you expect an implant to do better?

Everything we do has a limit on how long it can last before it needs to be adjusted, replaced or redone. Why? Wear and tear. Our mouths go through large temperature changes, bite changes, grinding, clenching, food getting stuck, trauma and so much more. Imagine getting a car and never taking care of it, never taking it for oil changes or regular maintenance. How long would you expect that car to last? Not very long! The same applies to your dental work.

- Fillings treat tooth decay. They can last anywhere from 3 to 10 years depending on

- many factors. I've seen some last 1 year and some in place for 12 years.

- Crowns fully cover a tooth that is broken, cracked or heavily decayed. Veneers cover only the front surface of teeth and are used to improve their appearance. Both can last for 10-15 years but I have seen some as short as 3 years and some longer than 20 years. If they do fail, it is often a result of a cavity forming in the area where the crown/veneer

- and natural tooth meet.

- Bridges replace missing teeth. It consists of one or more crowns that are fused together on top of a porcelain or metal base. The bridge is supported on either side by natural teeth. They typically last 7-10 years. Again, I've seen some as short as 3 years and some longer than 20 years. A bridge requires filing down the teeth adjacent to the missing tooth/teeth, which raises the risk of decay and/or damage in the teeth that support the

- crown.
- Nightguards can last 3-5 years depending on your grinding/clenching habit.
- Dentures can either replace an entire arch of teeth (top or bottom) or several missing teeth. They can last 5-10 years. The main factor is bone and gum atrophy as well as wearing out the acrylic. Sometimes a "reline" on your denture can make it fit properly
- again. Other times, an entirely new denture will need to be made.
- Implants also replace missing teeth. The implant itself is a post which is implanted into the bone and serves as a tooth "root". An abutment is attached to the post to support a dental crown. It is more difficult to set a range for implants. Typically, 10 years is the standard that implants are evaluated on. I've seen some last less than this and some still in the mouth for 25 years.

Regardless of the type of dental work, longevity is dependent on many factors including your bone, gums, oral hygiene, medical history, bite and clenching/grinding habits. Regular dental cleanings and checkups are essential to help extend the life of any dental work.

Cavities

"How often do you brush and floss? When was the last time you flossed?"

These are two of the most common questions you are going to be asked when going to the dentist. In some offices you may even hear it at every visit. But why do we keep asking this question? To be honest, it is mostly rhetorical. We already know the answer based on what we see (cavities, plaque, gum disease etc.).

Cavities are pretty well understood by patients of all ages. Whether you're 6 or 76, cavities usually don't need any further explanation. But this can be both good and bad. It is good that it is part of general knowledge and is accepted by everyone. It can also be bad if people don't really understand cavities. Sadly, there is a tendency (from patients and dental professionals alike) to focus on the treatment more than the actual problem. If we don't understand and treat the source of the problem, then things will tend to repeat themselves. This often leads to frustration for both the patient and the dentist. If I take an Advil or any other pain killer because I am not feeling well, that pain killer does not cure the problem, it simply masks the symptoms. It's a Band-Aid fix. It doesn't address the reason *why* we're not feeling well. The same is true with dentistry. This is why is important to understand the causes of tooth decay so you can learn how to properly care for your teeth and your health.

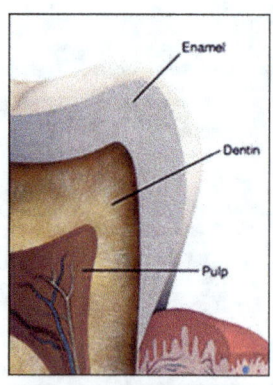

Figure 10: Layers of a tooth

So, what exactly is a cavity? Simply put, a cavity is the breakdown of your tooth by acid attack caused by bacteria. To fully understand what a cavity is, we need to understand the different layers of the tooth because cavities can spread. As seen in Figure 10 (Taken from Dental Care, 7), a tooth is composed of 3 main layers: the outer enamel, the inner dentin and the nerve or pulp tissue. Our outer enamel is harder than bone and small cavities that are only in enamel can sometimes reverse themselves, if we take the appropriate measures. At this point, it may not need a filling to reverse the damage. The next layer is dentin which is softer and usually leads to sensitivity if exposed or if the cavity spreads this far. When a cavity reaches the dentin, you need a filling because the cavity can no longer stop on its own. And finally, we have the nerve and blood vessels. If the cavity spreads to this level, you would require a root canal. A root canal removes all the nerve and blood vessels that are infected or dying off and seals the area where the nerve once was so you can keep your tooth.

Now that we know what a cavity is, what causes them and how do they spread or get larger? Cavities are caused by a combination of factors: bacteria in your mouth, frequent snacking, sipping sugary drinks and not cleaning your teeth well. Bacteria naturally live in your mouth and on your teeth. If these bacteria are not removed regularly, plaque forms and adheres to your teeth. When sugar combines with plaque, it produces acid which attacks the enamel of your tooth. The more sugar you consume, the more acid that gets produced. Over time, this can cause holes to form in your teeth, otherwise known as cavities. If left untreated, these holes can grow larger over time and can even destroy the entire tooth.

Cavities can develop in between the teeth, on the chewing surfaces (deep grooves), on smooth surfaces of the teeth and also on the surface of a tooth's roots. Cavities between the teeth occur when bacteria from food is not removed with flossing. You can also get cavities in the deep crevices and grooves on the chewing surfaces of teeth. Some people have deeper and steeper grooves where toothbrush bristles are not able to fully penetrate so bacteria and food get stuck in these areas and lead to decay. This is typically the case in adult molars. Sealants are often a good idea especially at an early age to help seal these deep grooves which make it easier for us to maintain ourselves through regular brushing. Smooth-surface cavities affect the flat exterior surface of teeth. These are the slowest of the cavities to develop and also the least common because our tongue and toothbrush have easy access to wipe and clean away any food or bacteria from these areas. Root cavities develop when gums recede and the root surfaces of a tooth become exposed, leaving it vulnerable to acid attack. It is very important to treat root cavities as soon as possible since decay in this area can spread quickly as this portion of the tooth does not have as much protective enamel.

Another question I often get asked is why some people get cavities and some don't. There are many factors that play a role. Some medications and medical conditions can promote tooth decay by changing the makeup and production of saliva. Saliva is protective because it helps wash away plaque from the teeth and buffer the acid. It also brings minerals that help repair teeth. A decrease in saliva production is referred to as "dry mouth". This condition allows plaque and bacteria to build up more quickly, making you more susceptible to tooth decay. Another factor is fluoride. Fluoride helps to protect teeth and make them more resistant to acid attack. Early use of fluoride as a child has been proven to have long-term benefits. Genetics also play a role. Some people simply have stronger teeth or teeth that are more capable of sustaining stress without reaching a point of a cavity, while others do not. Lastly, oral hygiene and education as well as parental attitudes toward dental care are often passed down from generation to generation. We could write an entire book about the different factors involved. The main point is education and frequent dental visits from an early age so we can determine where you fall in all of the factors listed above.

To give you an idea of how tooth decay will spread in a tooth, I've attached some x-rays of how a typical cavity will spread through a tooth if left untreated (Taken from Science Direct, 8).

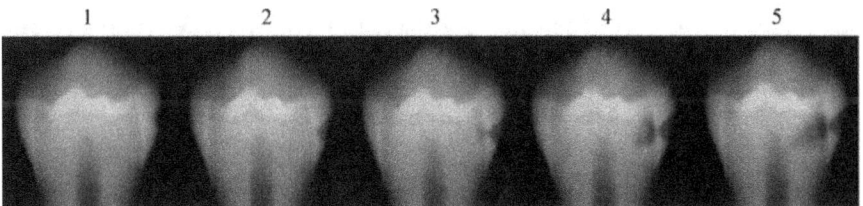

Figure 11: Tooth Decay Progression

Figure 11 was taken from an article that looked at when dentists decide to treat decay. This is not meant as an exercise for you to be able to read x-rays. It is simply a representation to show you how things spread. As you can see, decay is spreading from the outer enamel layers in 1 and 2 into dentin in 3 and 4 and finally into the nerve in 5. Now an x-ray only gives us part of the picture. Decay is usually even deeper than what we can see in the x-ray and is most likely spreading to dentin in picture 2.

In picture 1, we would usually monitor this lesion as long as it is stable upon clinical examination. Early cavities such as these can also be referred to as incipient decay. With proper oral hygiene (flossing, brushing and fluoride-containing rinses), these early cavities can reverse and won't need to be drilled and filled. It is always preferable to let the body heal on its own before drilling into a tooth if we have that as an option. At follow up appointments, we compare if there are any changes. If it looks the same or better then it is usually a good sign. If it looks worse (more like picture 2) or is causing pain and sensitivity, you are likely going to need a filling to reverse the damage. I would rather you get a filling at picture 2 or before picture 3. Once decay spreads into dentin, it can spread very quickly. At picture 5 the decay is very deep and most likely is into the nerve so you will probably need a root canal, a large filling and even a crown if the destruction is significant enough. This is another reason why early detection is very important. Sometimes it can take years for a cavity to spread through enamel and sometimes it takes less than a year depending on many of the factors we discussed earlier.

While it is best to avoid getting them altogether, cavities are fairly simple to treat. The most common treatment for a cavity is a filling, which is when the decayed portion of the tooth is drilled away and replaced with a strong filling made from amalgam, composite, glass ceramics, bioceramics or a combination. The choice of material will depend on the clinical situation and your preference. Treatment for more extensive decay can include crowns and root canals.

Now that you have fixed the cavity, you're all good, right? Unfortunately not. This is because once you have a filling or a crown, you can still get new cavities forming around any tooth replacement material. Let's think of a filling or crown like a vase that had a broken piece glued back to it. Even though the vase is whole again, there will always be a layer of glue between the broken piece and the original vase. The same principle applies to teeth. There will always be an interface between the tooth and filling material or crown that is susceptible to breakdown. We try our best with technology to make this as small as possible but it still exists. It can break down and bacteria can infiltrate and again cause destruction of the tooth from the inside. This is when we need to replace the filling/crown and create a new interface. This is the constant battle we face.

What is the lesson from all this? Avoid getting a cavity in the first place. By being preventative and taking care of your teeth, they are more likely to last much longer.

Crowns and Veneers

"I want to get veneers and look like Julia Roberts!"

Crowns and veneers are commonly confused with one another. They are often referred to as cosmetic and aesthetic dentistry. But are they? Well, yes and no - everyone's favourite answer.

Crowns are full coverage restorations (meaning they cover the entire tooth). They are indicated for many reasons including fractured teeth that can no longer be made whole by a filling, root canalled teeth that need stronger protection, cosmetic correction, teeth that are worn into the dentin, fixing the bite and more. They can be made the same day in the office but are more often sent to a dental lab for fabrication. They are commonly made of metal (stainless steel or gold), porcelain ceramics (Zirconia, Emax) or a combination of the two. Crowns are either cemented or bonded to the tooth.

Veneers cover only the front surface of a tooth (think of them as half-crowns). They are made of porcelain and are mostly used for cosmetic or for full mouth rehabilitation when we are changing or correcting your bite. These are typically what celebrities will receive to achieve that Hollywood smile.

On average, crowns and veneers can last 10-15 years but I have seen some as short as 3 years and some longer than 30 years. The life span of a crown/veneer can depend on the amount of "wear and tear" it is subjected to, oral hygiene practices and mouth-related habits such as clenching/grinding, biting fingernails, chewing ice, etc.

You cannot tell the difference between a crown and a veneer just by looking at someone's smile. However, the preparation and the restoration are different. They also provide different structural support and the choice between the two will depend on your clinical situation.

Figure 12 shows a case with 8 anterior porcelain veneers.

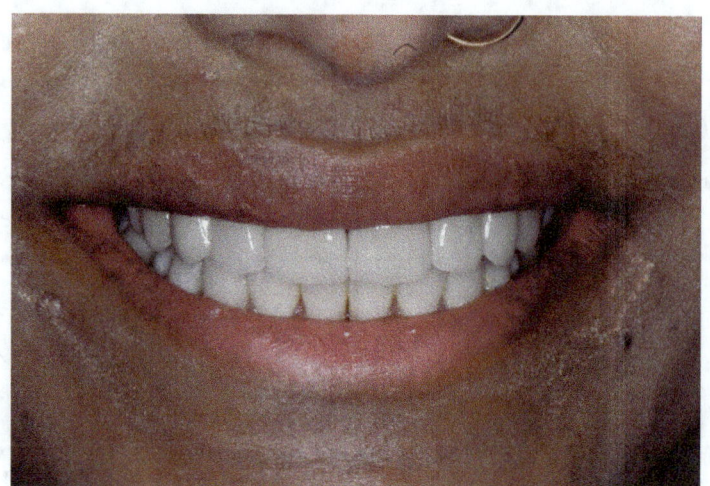

Figure 12: 8 Anterior Porcelain Veneers

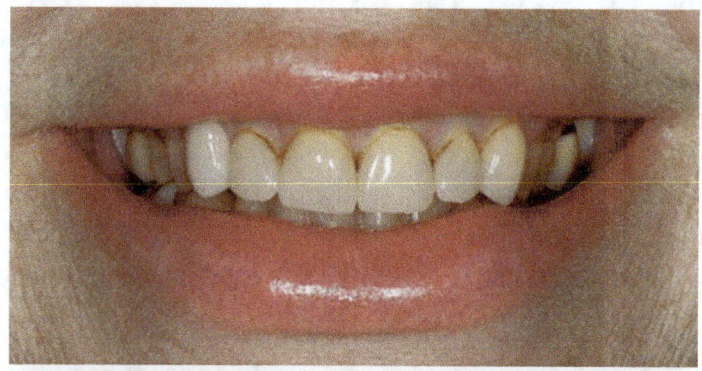

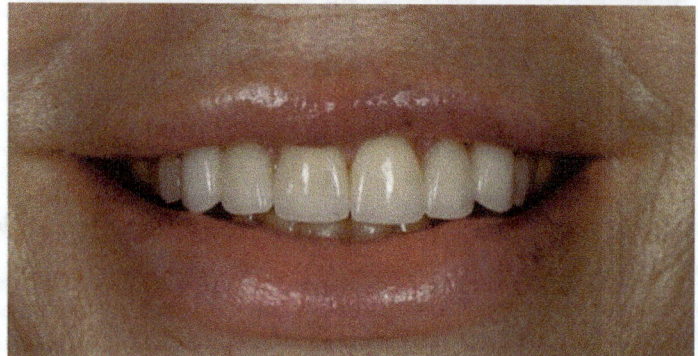

Figure 13: Before and after 8 porcelain crowns

Figure 13 is a before and after case of mine where we replaced some old veneers with 8 porcelain crowns. Both crowns and veneers do not stain and cannot be whitened, however the interface between the porcelain and the tooth can pick up stain and this is where failure can occur.

You will typically have two visits to the dentist for a lab-fabricated crown/veneer. At the first appointment, the tooth is "prepped". This means filing it down (across the top and sides for a crown and across the front surface for a veneer) to make space for the crown/veneer to fit snugly overtop. The amount of tooth that gets filed down will depend on many variables including what the final material will be, are we changing the colour or position and more. A putty is then used to take an impression (make a copy) of the tooth. An impression is also taken of the opposing teeth to ensure that your new crown/veneer will not affect your bite. The impression is sent to a dental lab for fabrication of the final crown/veneer which usually takes about a week. A temporary crown/veneer is made to cover and protect the "prepped" tooth while you wait for the permanent restoration. A temporary will also give you an idea of what the final result will look like in terms of colour, shape, contour and bite. This is the best time to pick out any changes or adjustments you want in the finals. Keep in mind that the material we use for temporaries have limitations and they won't look or feel as good as the finals. Be very careful with temporaries because they are mostly held in by friction and can break very easily. We do not want to permanently cement the temporaries because they can be very difficult to remove and this can affect the fit of the final restorations. At the second appointment, the temporary is removed and the fit and colour of the permanent crown/veneer is checked. If everything is fine, the new crown/veneer is permanently bonded in place using a dental cement.

Dental crowns can also be made in one visit with computer-aided design/computer-aided manufacturing (CAD/CAM) technology, if your dentist has the equipment. The initial process is the same – "prepping" the tooth. A scanning wand is then used to take digital photos of the prepped tooth. The computer's software will then create a 3D model of the tooth from these pictures. The crown is digitally designed and milled out of a ceramic block. The milling process takes about 15 minutes and the crown is then ready to be cemented.

So, when do you need crown? Crowns are usually indicated when teeth have root canals, large existing fillings that are covering a large part of the tooth, fractures and anatomic differences. Root canals will be discussed a little later but in its simplest terms, a root canal is essentially a hollowing out of your tooth to remove the infected nerve and infection. Once a tooth has had a root canal, it can become more brittle and prone to fracture because it is no longer alive (it no longer receives a blood supply). That is why it is a good idea to protect it with a crown. You want a good seal on the tooth so bacteria can't come back and cause re-infection. The best root canal with a bad filling will probably fail whereas a less than ideal root canal with a perfect crown will most likely be successful.

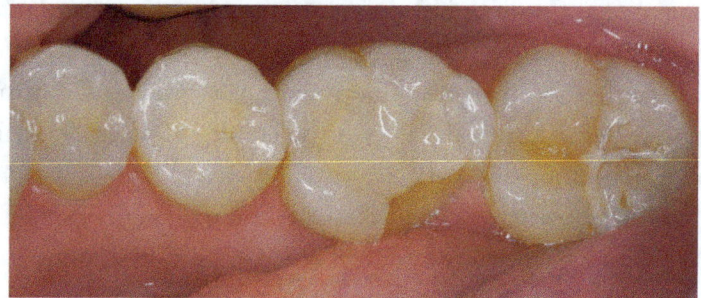

Figure 14: Fractured Molar

Fillings, like most things, have a limitation on how big they can get. You cannot replace an entire tooth with a filling because the bond won't be very strong. A filling relies on the remaining tooth structure to be successfully held in place. Once a filling reaches this limit, it can act like a wedge on the tooth and can cause fractures on the remaining parts of the tooth. Once this limit is reached, it is better to place a crown on the tooth instead of waiting for the tooth to fracture or replacing it with an even larger filling. In Figure 14, you can see a fractured molar where the large filling caused the inside part of the tooth to break off. It usually takes the path of least resistance to break the pressure. These situations can be avoided with crowns which move the outward pressure on these teeth back vertically toward the root.

A crown/veneer does not require any special care. However, the underlying tooth is still subject to decay and gum disease. It is important to floss daily, especially around the crown/veneer area where the gums meet the tooth.

Whitening

"Why can't I just whiten my teeth?"

Everyone wants a whiter smile. Even patients who come in with a list of pressing dental issues will want to address how to whiten their teeth first. Whitening has come to the forefront with everyone working from home on different virtual platforms. In essence, we are seeing what we look like for the first time. Normally, we would do a quick check on our appearance in a mirror throughout the day but when we are on a Zoom call we actually tend to look at ourselves rather than the other person. So, we start to notice things that we may have overlooked with a quick glance in the mirror.

Tooth whitening refers to any process that lightens the colour of teeth. The desire for whiter teeth is partly due to electronic, print and social media influences portraying perfectly white smiles. We see charcoal toothpastes, whitening toothpastes, fancy UV lights, lasers and celebrities swearing by any and all these products. With all the different options out there, how can you tell what will work and what won't? Basically, they all work to some extent – it just depends on your expectations and what colour you are starting with.

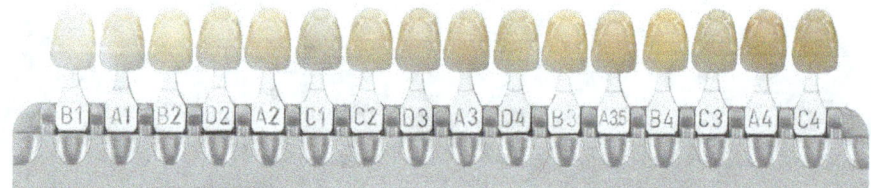

Figure 15: Traditional Vita shade guide - Lightest to darkest

Figure 15 shows a traditional Vita shade guide from lightest (B1) to darkest (C4). This guide is used by most dentists and dental companies to determine tooth shades as well as shades for restorative materials like fillings and crowns. It is also used to determine a before and after colour for in-office whitening. Generally, the higher you are on the shade guide (more left), the harder it is to upgrade to the next colour. There are colours beyond B1 where you start to get into bleach shades, however those colours are not very natural and teeth are not made to look that white. The natural colour of teeth ranges from light greyish-yellow.

Before you try any type of whitening, consult with your dentist or health care professional to make sure it is safe and will work for you. Not everyone will see results with teeth whitening. Typically, whitening works best for people with yellow teeth. It is less effective for people with brown teeth and probably won't work at all if your teeth have a gray tone.

Before we take a closer look at whitening, let's talk about staining. There are two types of staining – intrinsic and extrinsic. It is important to understand the difference because whitening can only improve extrinsic stains that occur on the surface layers of the tooth. Intrinsic stains involve the internal structure and development of the tooth and can be due to many factors such as genetics, early antibiotic use (tetracycline) during tooth development and the nerve of a tooth dying. Whitening unfortunately cannot undo any developmental changes of a tooth. Intrinsic stains will require restorative work to mask the staining or in the case of a root canalled tooth, will require internal bleaching.

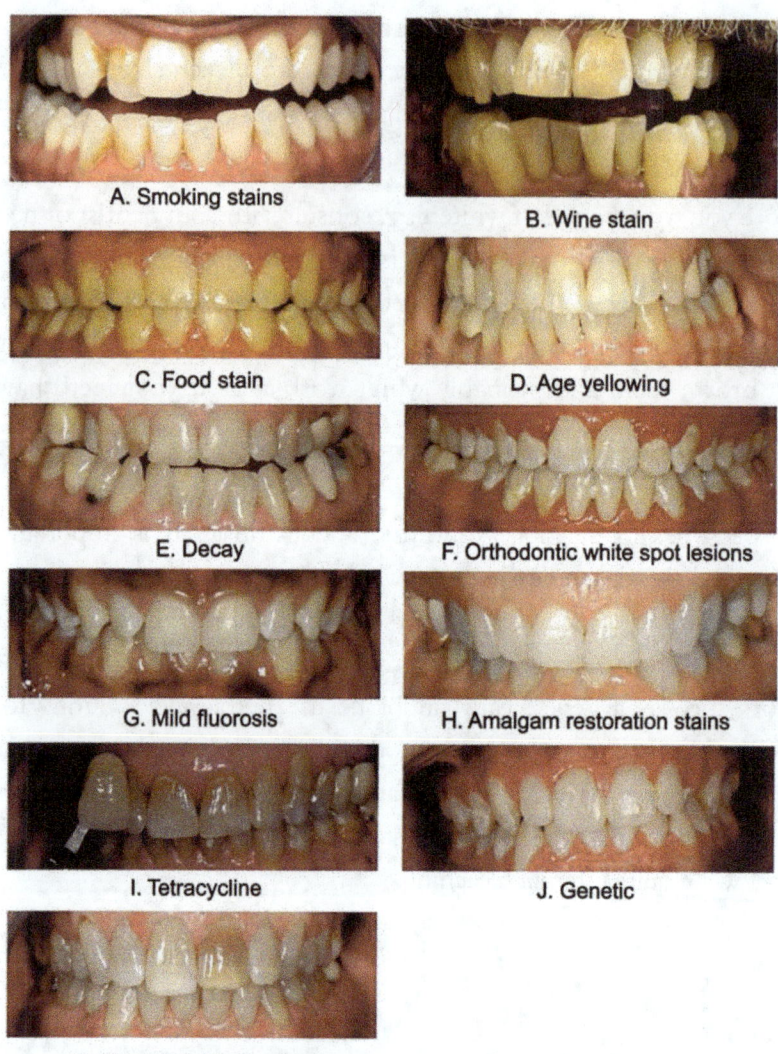

Figure 16: Different types of tooth staining

Extrinsic stains (or surface stains) are superficial discolouration involving the outermost layer of a tooth, or the enamel. The outer surfaces of teeth have pores and these pores are susceptible to staining from pigments in dark coloured foods, wine, tea, coffee, smoking etc. *(see Figure 16 – taken from Tooth Whitening, 9).* What whitening does is open up and clear out these pores so that these stains are no longer contributing to the overall colour of the tooth. However, once those pores open, they can cause sensitivity since those pores lead directly into the tooth and anything cold, sweet or even room temperature air can be uncomfortable until those pores close up again. They can be closed with certain toothpastes so that the staining is less likely to happen again or as quickly.

Teeth whitening can be professionally done in a dental office (in-office whitening) or at home (custom-made whitening trays, whitening strips or gels, toothpastes). Both options use peroxide-based agents: hydrogen peroxide or carbamide peroxide. Hydrogen peroxide is the actual bleaching agent, while carbamide peroxide breaks down into hydrogen peroxide. The concentration will differ if it's over-the-counter or available in the dental office. In-office whitening with a dental professional will use a much higher concentration so it has to be monitored because it can damage your gums if it is not applied correctly. This higher concentration can also lead to increased sensitivity compared to at-home whitening. Generally, the best approach is to do in-office whitening with at-home touch ups every few months to maintain the colour. When you utilize in-office whitening, your teeth will initially appear extremely white because your teeth are dehydrated. The colour will fade over the next few days as your teeth rehydrate. In-office whitening is generally safe as long as it is not done too often but make sure to check with your dentist to determine what the best regiment is for you.

And what about UV lights and lasers? Do they make teeth whitening faster and better? Unfortunately, there is no research to support any benefit from using UV lights or lasers in combination with teeth whitening. They are more of a marketing gimmick and that includes UV lights used for any in-office whitening as well. The active ingredient in the whitening gel is what makes your teeth whiter. But the light definitely makes a better social media post. Whitening toothpastes have become very popular in the last decade. We usually buy them without giving it a second thought. But are they actually good for your teeth? Whitening toothpastes fall into two categories – those that use abrasives (silica, baking soda, activated charcoal, etc.) to help remove surface stains and those that contain a bleaching agent. Most whitening toothpastes can only get your teeth about one shade lighter. You should not use whitening toothpastes more often than the label indicates as it can lead to teeth and gum sensitivity. In addition, persistent use can damage your tooth enamel and dental restorations (crowns, veneers, fillings) over time.

Charcoal toothpastes were heavily marketed in social media a few years ago. I would be very careful using them because they are too abrasive for everyday use and can wear out your outer enamel. And once you remove enamel, it does not come back. So why are charcoal toothpastes popular? The reason is that in the process of wearing down your enamel layers, they will also remove any superficial staining in those outer layers, which means your teeth will initially look whiter. However, prolonged use can in fact have the opposite effect. Teeth may eventually look yellower because as you start to thin out your enamel, you will expose the dentin which is naturally yellow. Loss of enamel can also lead to increased sensitivity and susceptibility to decay.

Charcoal toothpastes (and basically any toothpaste) have an abrasive rating to tell you how harsh they are. This abrasiveness is measured by the toothpaste's ability to cut dentin (the layer of teeth below enamel) and is scored as a Relative Dentin Abrasivity (RDA) value. This scale assigns toothpastes a value from 0 to 250. According to ADA standards, anything under 250 is consider safe for daily use and anything above 250 is considered a potential hazard to your enamel, with no degrees of safety between 0 and 250 on the RDA scale. Basically this means that a toothpaste ranked at 249 is equally as safe as a toothpaste with a ranking of 1. Although this is the underlying premise, I would still caution against long-term use of any whitening toothpaste as they are generally more abrasive. If you plan on using any charcoal or whitening toothpaste, make sure to look for one that has the lowest RDA value possible.

If you are considering using any whitening product, always consult with your dentist first to devise a plan that works for you. Your dentist will also let you know if you have any conditions that will not respond well to whitening or which may be aggravated by it.

Gum Recession

Gum recession is the physical drifting of the gum level away from a tooth. It drifts up on the upper teeth and down on the lower teeth. It can be caused by grinding, clenching, acid wear, an unstable bite, aggressive brushing and age, to name a few.

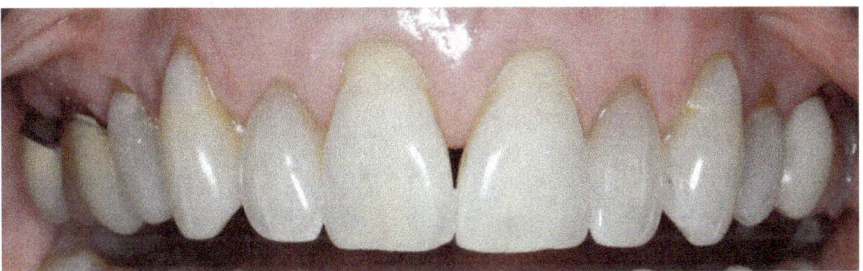

Figure 17: Gum recession on upper teeth

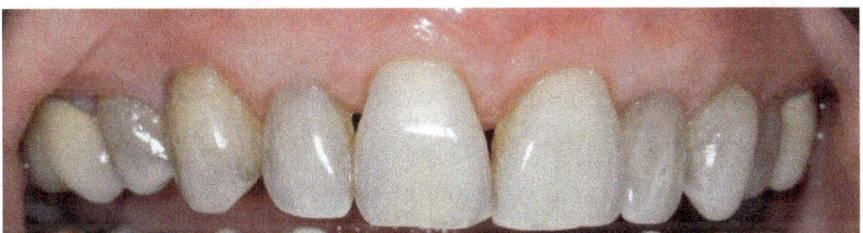

Figure 18: Post treatment of gum recession

In Figure 17, you can see generalized gum recession on the upper teeth caused by a bite issue which led to overnight clenching spanning many years. Figure 18 is the same patient after surgical treatment. As you can see, we have reversed most of the gum recession in all of the upper teeth. While surgery can correct the problem, it is important to understand the reason behind the gum recession before we treat it otherwise it will relapse and happen again.

So where does it all begin and how do you get gum recession? If you look at your teeth, what you see is only about half of what the entire tooth looks like. A large portion of your teeth is actually within your gum tissue and jawbone to anchor them in place. Over time, the gum tissue surrounding your teeth can begin to pull away and expose more of the surface area of the teeth. When this occurs, it is called "gum recession". The most common cause of gum recession is periodontal disease or gum disease. This happens when plaque builds up and bacteria attack the supporting gum tissue causing it to break down and recede from the teeth. Plaque build-up is the result of ineffective or infrequent brushing and flossing. Lifestyle choices such as smoking and use of tobacco products can also increase your plaque build-up, making it more difficult to effectively clean and remove bacteria from your mouth. Gum recession can also be a result of hormonal changes in the body from natural aging or from certain medications. Lastly, frequent grinding or clenching (particularly during sleep) can put undue strain and stress on the gums and jaw which can also lead to gum recession.

When gums start to recede, we often see different patterns of wear on the teeth like abrasions, abfractions and erosion. They all have varying causes and all involve some tooth damage but at different areas on the tooth. They can interact and it is possible to have all three at the same time.

So, what is the difference between abrasions, abfractions and erosion?

Abrasions

Abrasion is tooth wear resulting from friction from foreign objects (pens, fingernails, mouth piercings) or mechanical irritation (brushing too aggressively, using a hard-bristled toothbrush or abrasive tooth products). Tooth abrasion takes a long time so you may not even realize that it is happening at first. So, why is abrasion a problem? Over time, notches may develop near the gum line because the enamel has worn down and made the inner layers of the tooth more visible. When this happens, the enamel starts to wear out and the damage is usually consistent and continuous. Without the enamel, your teeth become more vulnerable to bacteria and plaque. You may also develop sensitivity to hot, cold, sweet or sour foods. Enamel cannot repair itself once it is damaged so be gentle when brushing, use a non-abrasive toothpaste and a soft-bristled toothbrush. In addition, try to break any bad habits like nail biting.

Abfractions

An abfraction is a notched out area on the root of a tooth at the gumline. It is caused by stress and pressure on the tooth and gums which results in breakage at the neck of the tooth. The hard enamel of the tooth is unaffected while the softer root becomes worn, which creates a notch at the gumline of the tooth. Over time, notched areas can deepen due to flexure, which occurs when teeth flex slightly at the gumline, causing it to slowly chip away – this happens with chewing, clenching and grinding. If left untreated, the notched areas can slowly deepen and can even affect the nerve of the tooth. When a tooth has an abfraction, it is likely to have abrasion as well because once dentin is exposed it wears a lot easier so sometimes they can be combinations. Figure 19 is a good example of tooth abrasion with abfractions. As previously mentioned you can see that the wear is continuous, of the same severity and in all the teeth. You can visualize the horizontal brushing motion that lead to this amount of damage. Abfractions are typically treated by filling in the notches with a composite material (basically doing a filling). A nightguard may also be recommended. If your bite is the underlying cause, you may want to consider orthodontics.

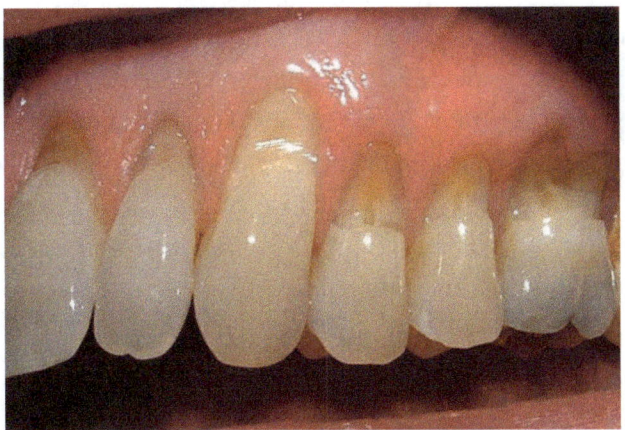

Figure 19: Tooth abrasion and abfractions

Erosion

Erosion is the general loss of tooth enamel due to acid attack. Exposing your teeth to acid can leach calcium from your enamel, causing it to break down. Acid can come foods and beverages you consume (e.g. wine, fruit juice, citrus fruits, candy, soft drinks, etc.). After consuming anything acidic, wait at least 30 minutes before you brush your teeth. Acid softens your enamel so brushing immediately after can actually cause damage. Saliva helps to wash acid out of the mouth so a reduction in saliva flow (dry mouth) can increase your risk of dental erosion. Vomiting and reflux can also cause stomach acids to enter your mouth and come into contact with the teeth. Unlike abfractions and abrasion, erosion occurs on the surface and subsurface of the teeth. If left untreated, erosion can lead to the progressive loss of the surface of the tooth, causing sensitivity, discolouration and even small cracks and dents. Once detected, it is very important to determine the cause to prevent further damage.

Now that we have outlined the possible outcomes from gum recession, what can you do to prevent it from happening in the first place? Prevention is always preferred because it is less invasive and less expensive. Orthodontics (either with braces or Invisalign) at an early age can help correct your bite. If your bite is stable then wear and tear will be less likely to occur. After orthodontics is completed, you will need retainers to prevent relapse otherwise the bite can destabilize again. If you find yourself clenching or grinding your teeth then a nightguard would be a good idea to help prevent any damage to both your teeth and gums. Over time if your bite changes, bite adjustments may be required to help re-stabilize your bite. If you lose a tooth then your bite can also change so always try to replace any lost teeth due to fractures or infection to make sure your bite remains stable.

But what happens if you already have gum recession? How do you fix it? Surgery is the only way to correct recession. There are many different methods that go beyond our short discussion here. Gum grafting involves taking tissue from another part of your mouth (usually the roof of your mouth) and placing it in deficient areas to help regrow or cover what has been lost. You can also use donated tissue and synthetics but your own tissue would give you the most predictable results. The success of gum grafting will depend on your medical history as well as your existing gum and bone levels prior to any corrective surgery. Although surgery will correct the recession, it is important to understand the reason why it happened in the first place so you can take the necessary steps to prevent it from happening again. Prior to gum grafting, fillings used to previously treat any abfractions will need to be removed because donated tissue can only attach to your tooth, not to filling material.

So why fix it? If you leave gum recession untreated, it can get progressively worse and will shorten the lifespan of your teeth. Recession exposes roots that are rough which trap more food and bacteria. This can lead to periodontal disease which leads to more recession and bone destruction and ultimately to the loss of your teeth. My treatment philosophy is for you to keep your teeth as long as possible because it has a direct link to quality of life and longevity as well. Elephants are very well known for this because once they lose their teeth, they are no longer able to take in the necessary nutrition they need and will pass away pretty soon after.

Nightguards

"But I don't clench or grind my teeth, why do I need a nightguard?!"

Nightguards have become increasingly common but what are they and do we really need them? Let's begin by looking at the problem they are meant to address – clenching and grinding. Clenching is the motion of biting down very hard and grinding is the action of biting down very hard and rubbing the teeth back and forth. Both are very common habits and usually occur when you are sleeping so you have no control over it and sometimes you don't even realize you are doing it at all. But why is it a problem? It's a problem because over time, you start to wear down your teeth. On average, our teeth touch cumulatively for about 9 minutes a day. This includes all the eating we do and even sometimes when we swallow. If you're grinding your teeth at night, chewing gum during the day or clenching your teeth while you're working out, this number can escalate very quickly. This force gets transferred to your muscles which in turn transfers it to your TMJ joints. All muscles in the body will grow the more you exercise them so the muscles in your cheeks, face and scalp will get bigger and stronger and thus transfer more force to your joint. This can lead to headaches, migraines, fractured teeth, broken fillings, lost crowns, fractured implants and more. Do I have your attention yet?

What causes us to grind or clench in the first place? There are many reasons why we grind or clench our teeth. Any mood-altering medications like antidepressants as well as recreational drugs can cause us to grind or clench our teeth. Medications that cause dry mouth can also make you grind in an effort to stimulate more saliva production. Another common reason though is stress. Stress can induce many anxious habits that we use as coping mechanisms to make us feel better. Biting our nails and chewing on a pen are just a few of the things we might start doing to help cope. Pain can also lead to grinding. When we have pain in the mouth, we tend to clench down as if we are trying to massage away the pain, much like a bruise on the outside of the body. Pain elsewhere in the body can also cause us to clench down. Think about what you do when you go through a painful event like putting an alcohol swab on a fresh wound – instinctively, you wince and clench.

The biggest factor, however, is your bite or how your teeth fit together. The topic of your bite (sometimes referred to as occlusion) is one that has many different theories and can be discussed at length. However, that is beyond what we are trying to do here. To put it as simply as possible, your bite is always changing. Your bite today is different than your bite 5 years ago and 5 years from now. Crazy, right? Our teeth are constantly undergoing stress, from daily events associated with eating and drinking (temperatures changes, acidity of our diet, etc.) and lifestyle habits such as smoking, drug use, medications and opening up things we shouldn't be with our teeth like beer bottles. In addition, as we age, our teeth slowly drift forward (known as mesial drift). And if you lose a tooth and don't replace it, all the other teeth start shifting and changing even quicker. So we are in a battle that we don't even know about and by the time we start to notice what is happening, so much has already changed.

What can we do then? First, we try to eliminate all the things that we can control. We start with changes such as altering our diet, stopping smoking, breaking bad habits and getting control of our health. Once we eliminate as much as possible then we can focus on your bite and how we can improve things. We cannot undo what has already been done in terms of any wear and tear however we can slow down the process and lower the frequency and severity of the habit. This is where night guards come in.

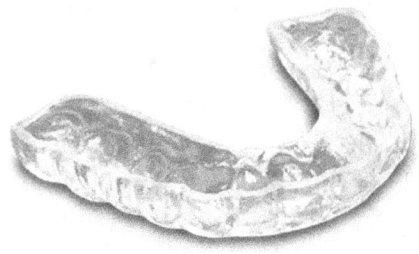

Figure 20: Nightguard appliance

There are two options when it comes to correcting your bite. The first is orthodontics (braces or Invisalign) which will be discussed in the next section. Orthodontics will place your bite in a stable position so you are less likely to grind/clench. If this is not an option, the next best thing is getting a nightguard. A nightguard is more of a Band-Aid fix because it only addresses the symptoms and not the root cause of grinding the teeth. A person who wears a night guard will usually continue to grind and clench their teeth. Nonetheless, a night guard is beneficial because it stabilizes your bite so it doesn't get worse. A nightguard also works as a barrier between your teeth and transfers the force from clenching and grinding away from your teeth so they don't get damaged.

What is a night guard? A night guard is a plastic dental appliance (Figure 20) that sits on top of your teeth. It can be made for your top teeth or for your bottom teeth. Sometimes it can be combined with a retainer depending on the clinical situation. I usually make them for the lower teeth because they tend to be more comfortable, they go with gravity and your tongue tends to accept it more than an upper. Night guards can be made with various materials but the goal is to cover your teeth as well as provide enough thickness to stabilize your bite and allow your muscles and joints to relax. You should get one that is custom made for your teeth and your bite. This can be done with your dentist. An impression will be taken of your teeth (top and bottom) to get a replica of your mouth and teeth. This is sent to a lab to create a night guard to fit precisely to your teeth. There are over the counter night guards but they are more for acute issues and trauma and should not be worn long term.

A night guard is worn at night when you sleep. Initially it may be difficult to get used to it. Habits are formed in 21 days so be persistent. Once you get used to wearing a night guard, you will feel like something is missing when you don't wear it! It is important to keep your night guard clean as it can trap bacteria and start to smell. If it smells, you are guaranteed not to wear it. To clean a night guard, rinse it with warm (not hot) water to remove any debris and prevent plaque from building up on it. Use a separate soft-bristled toothbrush and a mild antibacterial soap to brush it clean. Avoid toothpaste since it can be abrasive and damage the night guard. You can also soak it in a capful of mouth rinse diluted in water or an over the counter denture cleaner (fully submerge the night guard for about 30 minutes). Make sure to use an alcohol-free mouth rinse as alcohol can crack the acrylic over time. Let the night guard air dry completely before putting it back in its case to prevent bacteria from growing.

Night guards typically last 3-5 years depending on how much and how hard you are grinding and clenching. If you notice any chipping or cracks on the night guard, bring it to your dentist to have it assessed as this may indicate it is time for a new one.

Invisalign/Orthodontics

"Please tell me I don't need braces!"

As kids, we hear from our parents, our older siblings and other kids at school that eventually we'll need to get braces. But why do we need them? And why do we sometimes do it again later on in life?

It is a common desire to want straight teeth. But dentists will recommend orthodontics not because of aesthetics but because they want to correct the position of your teeth. It is an added bonus that putting your teeth in the correct position will also make them look nicer. Form will always follow function. If teeth are positioned where they should be then they will last longer, be easier to clean and be less likely to start wearing out and cause issues. Okay, so if I do braces then I'm done for the rest of my life, right? I never have to worry about my bite again? Wrong. This is why we get retainers once orthodontics is complete. Think of retainers as an insurance policy. We will always get relapse because of what we discussed in the last chapter in terms of mesial drift and the daily stress our teeth undergo. In addition, the ligaments around our teeth don't settle as fast as our teeth do and will try to move things back. Retainers maintain your bite as much as possible and slow this process down. However, life happens and we often forget to wear our retainers or they break and we don't get them replaced. So, our teeth start to shift again and we end up needing braces again later in life. But the idea of wearing metal braces as an adult is not very appealing. This is where Invisalign comes in. I will speak more about Invisalign because that is what I do in private practice but both Invisalign and braces work similarly and will get you the same result.

Invisalign has become increasing popular with people on Zoom and Facetime meetings looking at themselves 8 hours a day for the first time. Although there are other people on the video calls, instinctively you will look at yourself. And we start fixating on imperfections we want to change. And the first thing we notice is our smile.

But wait, how do I know if I'm a candidate for Invisalign? Bottom line, almost everyone is a candidate for Invisalign. 99% of cases that can be done with braces can now also be done with Invisalign. Invisalign can help correct crowding, close gaps, fix cross bites, widen your arches and correct a deep bite or an open bite. It can do it all. It can even be used in tandem with jaw surgery cases. And the technology gets better every day. Invisalign is even an option for children but compliance often becomes an issue so traditional braces may be a better choice, depending on the child.

What exactly is Invisalign and how does it work? Invisalign uses a series of clear plastic removable trays or aligners to slowly move teeth into position. The trays are customized for each patient using a 3D scan. Composite attachments are placed on the teeth to change the surface area of the tooth and provide anchorage to help move teeth. Elastics can also be used to create space in between the teeth to help correct crowding. Amazing, right? You can fix the position of your teeth by wearing these nearly invisible aligners and no one will even know that you are having orthodontic work done. As amazing as Invisalign is, it requires discipline. The success of any Invisalign treatment is dependent on patient compliance. In order to produce the best results, you need to wear the aligners for at least 22 hours a day - you only remove them to brush and floss your teeth and when you are eating or drinking anything other than water. Before putting your aligners back in after eating, it is imperative that you brush your teeth otherwise you increase your risk for cavities and bad breath. Food particles can also hinder tooth movement and can stain your aligners.

How long does Invisalign take to work? Well, it depends on your expectations and goals. We try to keep most Invisalign cases to under a year but sometimes it can take closer to 2 years. We can only go so fast when it comes to tooth movement. Going too fast can lead to root resorption (shortening of the roots) and that is not something anyone wants. So please listen to your dentist when it comes to the speed and duration of your case.

Figure 21 shows a before and after of an Invisalign case. This case took 9 months and addressed a few issues. The patient was concerned about her gums receding but the real issue was the bite that was causing the receding gums. By stabilizing the bite, we improved her smile and her chewing, made oral hygiene easier and stopped the receding gums. Once the bite was corrected, we could then surgically treat the receding gums with a high degree of certainty that the outcome would be predictable and less likely to relapse.

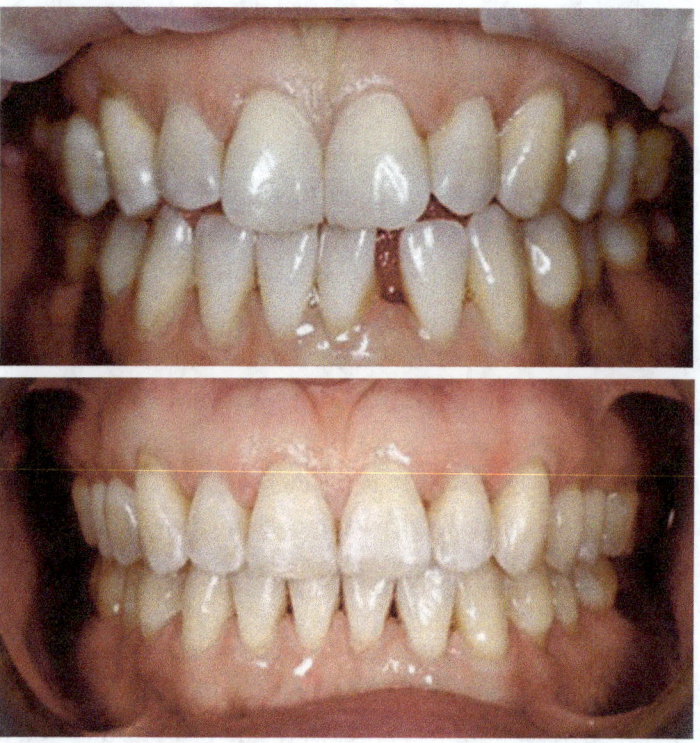

Figure 21: Invisalign treatment, before and after

Don't hesitate to gain the confidence and healthier life that a beautiful, straight smile can bring. Ask your dentist how orthodontics can help.

Extractions

"Alright, just yank it out!"

Other than root canals, extractions are probably the next dreaded thing that can happen at the dentist. While we do everything, we can to try to save a tooth, sometimes it's just not worth saving. Like the song goes, you have to know when to hold them and when to fold them. As children, baby teeth get pulled when they are infected or if they don't fall out in time. We even have a special character made for such occasions - the tooth fairy. The tooth fairy collects teeth and is willing to pay you for that extracted tooth. All you have to do is place it under your pillow before you go to sleep and you will be rewarded with cold hard cash in the morning. This can range from a few dollars to even $100 a tooth according to some stories. Not bad, right? Unfortunately, we all grow up to catch one of our parents swapping out our baby teeth for money (sorry if I ruined it for you). Usually by the time this happens, we run out of baby teeth to swap out so it all works out in the end.

Let's start at the beginning. Baby teeth get extracted when there is trauma, infection or fractures. Basically, we don't want any infection or trauma to spread to the adult teeth so extraction is a way to minimize any potential risk. Depending on the tooth and the age when it is taken out, a space maintainer may need to be made to prevent the surrounding teeth from shifting and covering the space necessary for the adult tooth to come in properly. If a baby tooth falls out, never try to put it back in – that's only for adult teeth. Also, never perform your own extractions at home even though it makes for a great social media video. You can damage the adult tooth underneath or leave a piece of the baby tooth behind if it breaks off. Extracting baby teeth is usually a simple procedure and most kids are back to normal the very next day.

Extraction of adult teeth is a little different. Like children, we take adult teeth out when there is infection or trauma. Another reason is impactions, when a tooth does not have enough room to develop or grow in properly, like wisdom teeth. However, before taking out an adult tooth we must consider how we are going to replace it. Why is this important? Think of your teeth as a row of books on a bookshelf - if you pull one book out, all the other books will start to collapse around the space. Neatly in a row, they keep each other lined up and stable. The same is true for your teeth. When a gap is left by a missing tooth, the surrounding teeth will shift to try and fill that gap. Over time, teeth may become crooked or new gaps may appear between teeth. Your bite will also shift and you will end up putting pressure on teeth that are not meant to handle more pressure. Super-eruption can also occur. This happens when a tooth grows out from its position because it no longer has an opposing tooth to resist it.

What are your options then for replacing a missing tooth? You can replace missing teeth with implants, bridges or partial dentures. You can also choose to do nothing but this should never be an option. Each option will have different risks and benefits but an implant is the closest thing to a natural tooth. Another important consideration when a tooth is extracted is grafting. When we remove an adult tooth, the gums and bone in that area will shrink because the body believes nothing is there so it doesn't waste any energy maintaining it. The body is very efficient in this regard. Without a graft, it can be harder to place an implant in the future or to clean the area properly if doing a bridge. To play it safe, always graft the area with a bone substitute regardless of how you are replacing the tooth in the future. When in doubt, graft. It is always easier and less expensive to preserve bone than to rebuild it in the future.

Wisdom teeth

What about third molars (wisdom teeth)? Everyone has heard dreaded stories of swelling up like a chipmunk, eating through a straw and funny YouTube videos of being sedated and saying all kinds of crazy things. Removing wisdom teeth, however, is a common occurrence and most people heal within 3-7 days.

Wisdom teeth can come in a variety of shapes, sizes and even numbers. Some people have no wisdom teeth and some people can have up to 7 of them. They are generally a remnant of evolution - we no longer need them based on changes in our diet and physiological changes (smaller jaws) mean there is hardly any room for them anymore. Impacted wisdom teeth can start pressing on the second molars, cause cavities, gum issues and infections. It is a good idea to start looking at removing them around 17 years old depending on their positioning and development – a panoramic x-ray will help us make this determination. Ideally you want to remove them before you turn 26 – beyond this, the procedure may be more difficult and the potential complications can increase. As well, the root development of lower wisdom teeth can get entangled with sections of the trigeminal nerve which could increase your chances of a nerve injury. It is preferable to remove a wisdom tooth earlier instead of waiting to see if the roots develop in that direction. Grafting after removal of wisdom teeth may be necessary if there is significant bone loss due to infection, cysts, gum disease or depending on proximity to the second molar.

Do I need sedation to take teeth out? It all depends on the person and the difficulty of the procedure. Unless we are removing one or two simple teeth, sedation is preferred to make the procedure more comfortable and safer. There are different levels of sedation - from minimal with laughing gas all the way up to a general anaesthesia. Your dentist will discuss the risks and benefits of each type of sedation so you can make an informed decision.

Root Canals

"Whatever you do, don't let them do a root canal."

Undoubtedly, root canals are one of the most-feared procedures at a dental office. Ask anyone and you will probably get the same reaction… the dreaded cringe. There are so many horror stories that get passed down from one generation to the next that some patients won't even consider saving a tooth with a root canal. But why do root canals have such a bad reputation? And are they really that bad?

To answer that question, let's quickly review our tooth anatomy. The outer part of the tooth is the white enamel and the layer underneath is the dentin. Inside each tooth is soft tissue that contains nerves and blood vessels. This is known as the pulp. The pulp extends down into the tooth's roots and supplies the blood that brings nutrients to keep the tooth alive. The thin channels housing the pulp are called the root canals. So, the term "root canal" refers both to the name of the procedure and also to the part of the tooth that's treated by it.

So, what is a root canal and when do we need one? A root canal is needed when the pulp inside a tooth becomes infected. The infection can stem from a deep cavity, trauma, bacteria introduced through a crack on the surface of the tooth or when gum infections spread to the bottom of the tooth. If left untreated, the infection can spread into the root canals of the tooth into the gums and form an abscess or swelling. Ideally we want to treat a tooth before an abscess forms because it will be harder to get you frozen. Sometimes it is better to use antibiotics first to bring the swelling/bacterial load down enough to freeze comfortably before proceeding with a root canal. Bear in mind that antibiotics will not cure the issue as the jaw has a poor blood supply and the antibiotics cannot get to the source of the infection which is inside the tooth. Once the antibiotics have left your system, the infection is likely to flare up again. Often, the pain that is mistakenly associated with a root canal is most likely the pain caused by the infection itself. What a root canal does is get rid of the infection. So, a root canal will make you feel better, not worse.

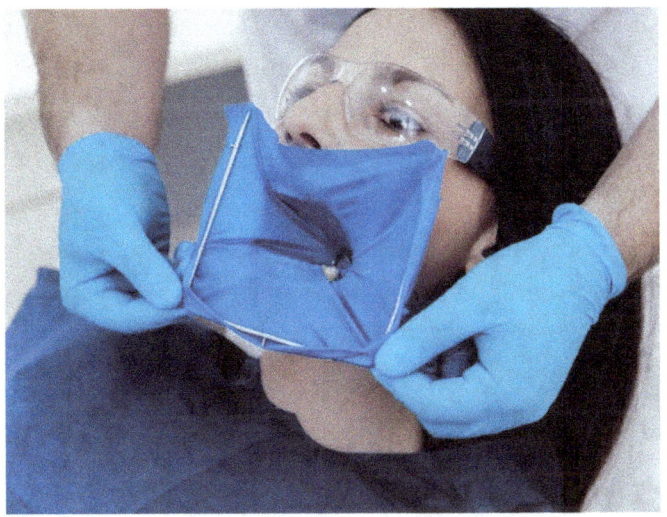

Figure 22: Rubber dam

The first step of a root canal is removing the infection. This is done by drilling into the infected tooth (after numbing you first, of course) and removing the diseased pulp. Once the pulp is removed, the root canals are cleaned out and disinfected and the now-empty space is filled with a clean inert material that prevents things from leaking back into the tooth. This is the most important step – creating a long-lasting seal. In order to do that, we need to prevent any new bacteria from reaching the internal chamber of the tooth. To keep the working area as sterile and dry as possible, a rubber dam is used to isolate the tooth receiving the root canal. All other teeth, gum tissues, cheeks, lips and tongue are protected underneath this barrier. This barrier essentially prevents your saliva (which contains bacteria) from contaminating the open tooth. It also keeps the materials used in a root canal from touching the inside of your mouth. Rubber dams may not be that comfortable, especially if you have a sensitive gag reflex or if you are claustrophobic, but they are used for your safety.

Root canals can be difficult, especially with molars, because the anatomy has so many variations and sometimes we are not able to find all the canals in a tooth. Remember, we are dealing with openings that are sometimes smaller than 0.1mm that can run in different directions and with possible calcifications blocking them. Since the majority of the root canal takes place within the hollow chamber of the tooth, including its roots, multiple x-rays will need to be taken throughout the procedure to ensure the correct positioning of tools and materials. This is all normal and a necessary part of the treatment.

What happens after a root canal? The process of a root canal essentially hollows out the tooth. Without the pulp, the tooth will become brittle and prone to fracture – basically, it's dead from the inside. A dental crown is the final step in many root canal treatments and is recommended to protect them from fracture. This is particularly true for back teeth (molars and premolars). These teeth bear the most force when biting and need the added strength of a crown. Other factors that determine whether a tooth will need a crown after root canal treatment include past tooth damage, clenching/grinding and patient oral health.

Okay, I had one root canal and now they're telling me I have to get another one for the same tooth? How many root canals am I going to have to go through? Yes, it's true. You may need another root canal on the same tooth in the future. This is referred to as a root canal retreatment. Basically, we re-enter the root canal, remove the filling and clean the canal(s) for a second time. But how and why does this happen? Studies show that initial root canal treatment has a success rate of 85-97%. However, root canals are a tricky business. If the infected tooth pulp is not thoroughly removed, the infection will essentially be sealed in the tooth, only to flare up later. Molar teeth typically have three canals, but sometimes a tooth can have a "hidden" fourth canal and sometimes a canal will branch out at a right angle. If there are any accessory nerve canals that we cannot get to due to complicated canal anatomy, if the placement of the crown is delayed or if something breaks and bacteria leaks into the tooth, the canal system can get infected again. Since you don't have nerves or blood vessels there, you really don't know until it's become significant. If retreatment is not a good option or does not solve the problem, endodontic surgery may still be able to save the tooth. The most common is an apicoectomy or root-end resection. This involves opening up the gum tissue near the tooth to see the underlying bone, remove any infected tissue and resection the end of the root. Your dentist will discuss all these options with you to help you make the best decision and give you the best long-term prognosis for your tooth.

Root canals really do not deserve the bad reputation that they have earned. Now that you know the what, why and how, let's remember to address the situation early, take antibiotics before, always get a crown after and get the courage to accept the rubber dam. That way we can tell our kids that root canals are not be feared.

Implants

"You're going to put a screw in my jaw? Are you serious?"

Dental implants have been around for close to 40 years yet most patients know very little about them. I believe they are the best treatment option to having a natural tooth again. So why don't people know more about them? I believe the blame goes both ways. From the perspective of the dentist, we sometimes don't spend as much time as we should educating our patients due to time constraints and scheduling. And from the patient view, you should always do your own research with guidance from your dental health professional so you can have as much information as possible. This is why education is so important. My hope is that after reading this chapter, everyone will be ready to talk about implants not only with their dentist but with their friends and family.

Implants have traditionally been made of titanium but recently a second player has been added to the game - ceramic implants. I will start the discussion with titanium because it has been around the longest and is the most well-known. We will discuss ceramic implants afterwards and look at why it was necessary to have a second option.

What is a dental implant? A dental implant is a post that is placed into your jawbone to serve as the foundation for a tooth. Implants in medicine don't last forever and need to be replaced at regular intervals, however in dentistry people have the belief that things last forever which is just not the case. If I'm replacing a tooth with an implant and that tooth did not last forever, why would you expect an implant which isn't as good as a natural tooth to last longer? It's just not going to happen. Implant longevity is usually evaluated at 10 years as the standard. I've seen some last for less than 5 years and some still in the mouth 25 years later. There are many factors that contribute to the long-term success of an implant. These include, but are not limited to, factors such as medical history (which can change after getting the implant), oral hygiene habits (which is different for implants), the surgery and site the implant was placed in, the type of implant used, your overall bite and grinding. We try to control as many of these variables as we can to make things more predictable but the more factors we have to fight against, the less likely we will win. Along the way, much like a tooth, the implant may need some revision to extend its longevity. This can mean a bone graft, gum graft or changing the crown. However, there will be a point where revision is not recommended and it would be better to remove the implant and start over. You have to know when to hold them and when to fold them.

Let's take a look now at the different stages involved in getting a dental implant. The best and most predictable method is an immediate implant - this occurs when we extract a tooth and place the implant the same day. A bone graft will also be done to cover the gaps where the tooth/roots were because the implant won't be as large as the roots/socket space. An immediate implant will save you time and money but more importantly, it will preserve as much of the bone and gums as possible. Sometimes we cannot place an immediate implant for anatomical reasons. In this case, we will graft the area after removing the tooth to maintain as much bone and gum as we can. After the graft heals (3-6 months), we will go back in and place the implant. Once the implant is placed, it will need to heal and integrate with your own bone to become one piece. This healing phase, which typically takes 3-6 months, is crucial to achieve a secure attachment. Now comes the second phase of the procedure. At this appointment, the implant will be exposed (a small incision is made in your gums), an abutment will be place on the implant and an impression will be taken to fit for a crown. The final step, which occurs about 2 weeks later, involves securing the crown to the implant.

Sometimes we secure a temporary tooth to the implant on the same day that it is placed, especially if it is a front tooth because we don't want you to walk around with a gap in the front during the healing phase. In order for this to happen, the implant needs to be really stable at surgery, the tooth needs to be out of your bite and you cannot chew on it. If you put pressure on the implant before it becomes stable, the cells around the implant will heal into gum tissue and not bone so the implant ultimately falls out. There are other methods of replacing the tooth while the implant heals that will not put as much pressure on it such as a removable denture, a clear retainer you can wear with a tooth in that missing spot or even a Maryland bridge that is cemented in to cover that area. Your dentist will review your options and decide what will be best for your case.

What if you are missing all of your teeth? Can you do implants for a full mouth? Absolutely. Full mouth implants refer to any implant procedure that replaces all of your missing teeth in either the upper or lower arch. This is usually done with two to six implants working together to support a full bridge or denture. The average denture has fourteen teeth on it. So, the more implants you have, the more stable the denture will be. Four implants is the best option for stability, but six would be even better. Treatment options for the upper and lower arch are basically the same, however additional implants are sometimes needed on the upper to compensate for softer bone.

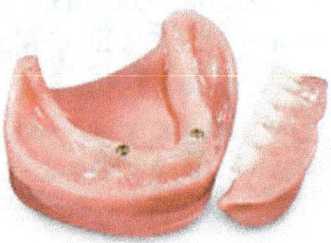

Figure 23: Removable overdenture

The most basic option uses two implants as anchors to support a removable denture that snaps in and out with ball attachments (Figure 23, taken from Glidewell, 10). This is common for lower dentures because there is no suction required for retention. The denture is held in place but it can still move in the back. Attachments and clips will periodically need to be replaced due to wear. Another option uses a custom-fitted bar attachment, which essentially splints the implants together, making them stronger. This support bar is affixed to four to six implants and the denture snaps into place using retention clips. This style is called an "overdenture".

Implants

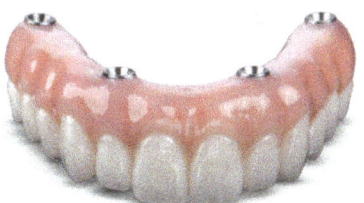

Figure 24: All on four hybrid

The more common option involves placing four to six implants and connecting a denture directly to these implants with screws on the day of the implant surgery (Figure 24, taken from Glidewell, 11). It's an amazing treatment option that works very well and is very predictable. However, because it is fixed (meaning you cannot remove it), oral hygiene is much tougher and you have to spend upwards of 20 minutes a day to properly clean underneath the fixed denture. This is an important factor in deciding which treatment option works best because if you don't commit to cleaning underneath the fixed appliance then it will cause a lot of issues. Some people will choose the removable denture option because of this.

Figure 25 is an All-on-6 case in the mouth so you can see how the fixed appliance looks visually. The materials we use for removable dentures has a limitation as to how lifelike they can be so when we transition to something fixed in the mouth, we are able to use other materials that allow us to come a lot closer to being lifelike. In the case below, we used Zirconia (a type of ceramic) in addition to staining for the colouring.

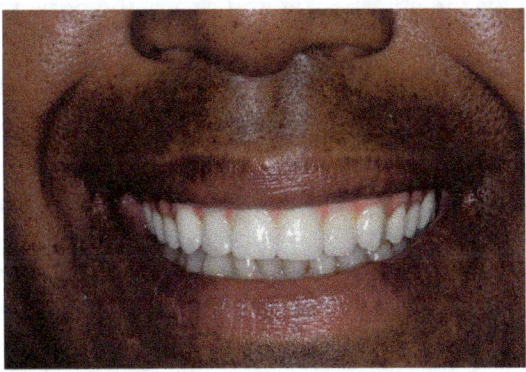

Figure 25: All on 6 Zirconia Final Hybrid

Oral hygiene for implants is extremely important. Just like natural teeth, plaque can collect on implant crowns and harbour bacteria. Remember that both natural teeth and dental implants rely on healthy supporting gums and bone for support. Proper oral hygiene can be very time consuming and the commitment needs to be there from day one, and if possible, before the implant treatment. Neglected implants develop plaque and tartar which can lead to peri-implantitis, an inflammatory condition that affects both the soft and hard tissues surrounding implants. If left untreated, bone loss can occur and lead to the implant becoming loose. Essentially, there are two parts to implant maintenance and success – regular checkups and cleaning by your dental team and your daily oral hygiene habits. How you care for your implant is critical to its overall health and long-term success.

Oral hygiene doesn't change all that much for implants but some of the details are different. The gum tissue that forms around an implant is different than the tissue around natural teeth. The connection is not as strong so the gums aren't as resilient. Even flossing the same way you would floss natural teeth can damage the gums around an implant. Use floss that won't shred or fray (avoid tufted floss or Superfloss) as floss particles can become stuck under the implant, which can increase the risk of infection or plaque build up around the implant. Flossing around dental implants should be done very gently – never push the floss down into the gum pocket. Aggressive flossing can break the protective seal created by the surrounding tissue around the implant. If the seal breaks, bacteria can enter the gum pocket and access the bone which supports the implant. Interproximal brushes (think of them as tiny toothbrushes) should be used to keep the spaces in between dental implants free of food and plaque. Make sure that it plastic-coated. Brushes with metal wires should be avoided as they can cause irritation to the soft tissue around an implant.

A Waterpik® is probably the best tool to use around implants, either as an adjunct to or in place of flossing. It loosens and flushes away plaque with a pressurized water stream. You can control the power of the device and use it at a lower setting around implants. Brushing is the same as you would brush natural teeth – use a soft-bristled manual toothbrush or an electric toothbrush. As always, it is best to brush twice daily – in the morning and before bed. For an All-on-x prosthesis, oral hygiene is the same as discussed above. The only additional consideration is that food particles can become trapped between the base of the denture and the gum line. Waterpik® has a special angled tip designed to direct water under an implant-retained denture. Lastly, toothpaste needs to be low-abrasive. Avoid toothpaste containing stannous fluoride, a higher concentration of sodium fluoride (>3.0), baking soda, stain removers, whitening agents and smoker's toothpaste. Natural teeth need a mild abrasive to polish the enamel but implants do not. Abrasives can scratch the surface of any exposed surfaces of the implant and can lead to future staining. Along the same line, avoid any type of teeth-whitening mouthwash or ones that contain alcohol as prolonged use can damage the acrylic.

Let's move on now to ceramic implants. What are ceramic implants and how are they different from titanium implants? Ceramic implants have been around since the early 2000's. They have been used in medicine for years but have been slow to gain traction in dentistry. They were developed not as a replacement for titanium implants but as an alternative in specific situations. One reason is patient sensitivities and allergies. Titanium implants are made of an alloy, which means that there is a mix of other metals, including nickel which is a common allergen. The titanium implant also has many different parts - you have the implant itself which is one titanium alloy, the abutment that screws into the implant (which could potentially be a different titanium alloy) and then a metal crown that either cement or screws into the abutment. In total, you potentially have 2-3 different metal alloys interacting with each other in the mouth with saliva. Studies have shown that this can lead to different interactions, corrosion, gum inflammation and other issues. All of this can be avoided with the use of ceramic implants. Ceramic implants are hypoallergenic. They are made using zirconia, a ceramic material made from zirconium oxide. The implant is completely white which means that it does not show through gum tissue, which is something that can happen with titanium implants if gum tissues thin over time or if recession occurs.

Ceramic implants are also bio-compatible – they are made from an inert, non-conductive and non-corrosive material. This means that they are less likely to attract and retain plaque and bacteria.

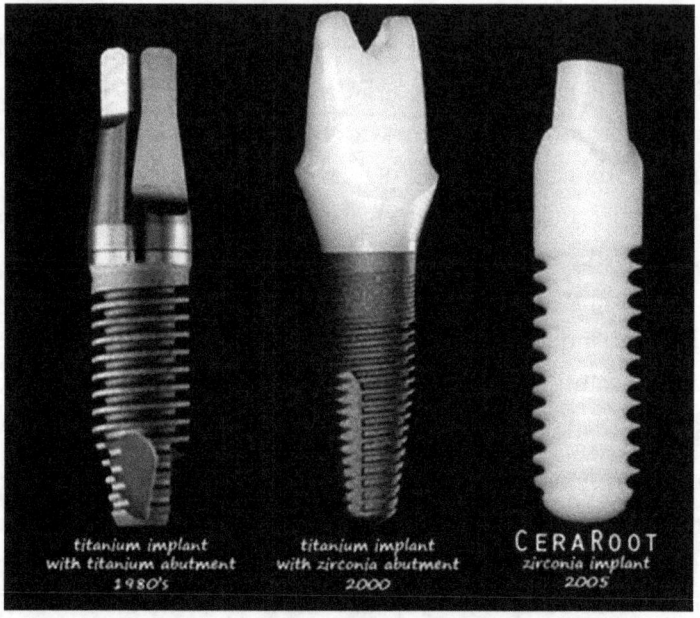

Figure 26: Titanium vs. Ceramic Implants

Figure 26 shows a titanium implant on the left, a ceramic implant on the far right and the evolution of how we got there with a hybrid in between (taken from www.ceraroot.com). CeraRoot has one of the longest track records and research available for ceramic implants and is a great resource for both dentists and patients when it comes to implant information. Ceramic implants are a relatively newer technology and as such the clinical indications they are used for are limited compared to titanium implants. Currently, ceramic implants are used for single tooth replacement and bridge cases. They cannot be used for full mouth rehabilitation or in areas that require a small diameter implant due to thin bone or small spaces between the teeth.

I place both titanium and ceramic implants. The choice is both clinical and patient-driven. I always present both options to patients, if applicable, so they can make an informed decision.

Figure 27 shows a ceramic implant case of mine where we placed an immediate CeraRoot implant and restored it with a ceramic crown.

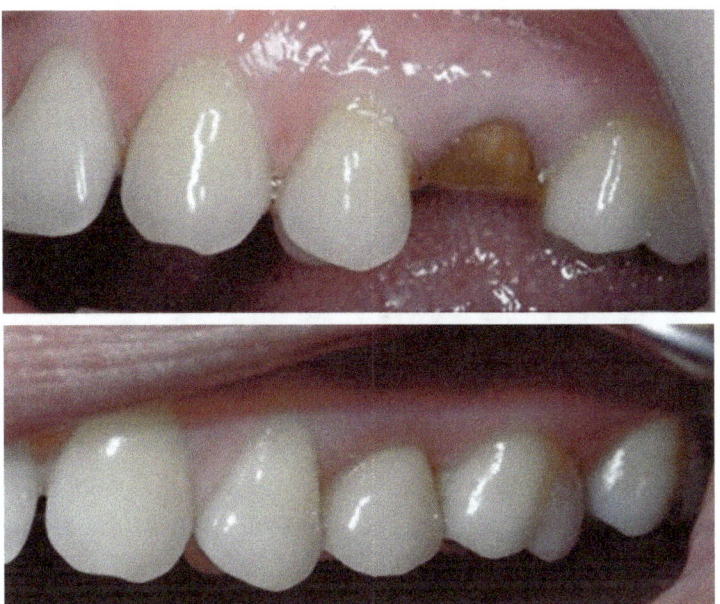

Figure 27: Before and after ceramic implant

Replacing a missing tooth or teeth is important for your oral health, which is tied to your overall health. If you are considering getting a dental implant, both ceramic and titanium implants are viable options. Each will offer a long-lasting solution. Consult with your dentist to find the material best suited for your personal situation.

Pregnancy

"I don't want to do anything to harm my baby. It's not safe to have a dental cleaning when I'm pregnant, right?"

This is one of the most common misconceptions in dentistry. Not only is it safe to have dental care during pregnancy, it is actually beneficial.

During pregnancy, it is not only your body that goes through changes. Increases in hormone levels can also change your oral health. Taking care of your teeth is important at any stage of your life, but it is especially important during pregnancy.

It is common for pregnant women to develop a condition known as "pregnancy gingivitis", an inflammation of the gums which can cause tenderness, swelling and bleeding when brushing or flossing. Although it is normal, it is important to make sure that you treat these symptoms – usually with more frequent cleanings. Left untreated, it can lead to periodontal disease (infection of the bone that holds the teeth in place) which can have serious repercussions.

Pregnant women may be more susceptible to cavities due to changes in diet and frequent snacking. Despite cravings, be sure to monitor sugar intake. Severe or prolonged morning sickness can also cause acid erosion of the teeth. Pregnant women should avoid brushing their teeth immediately after vomiting. It is best to wait at least 30 minutes before brushing. It is a good idea to rinse with a baking soda solution (one cup water to one teaspoon of baking soda) after vomiting to neutralize the acid. Although rare, pregnancy hormones can cause benign growths in the mouth. These are not dangerous and usually disappear after delivery. If you are concerned, talk to your dentist about having them removed.

You may not realize it but a baby's teeth start to develop during the second and third trimester. It is important that pregnant women maintain a healthy diet to support healthy teeth development in their babies. In addition, bacteria that cause cavities can be passed to your baby during pregnancy and after birth.

Be sure to let your dental office know that you are pregnant, or if you trying to get pregnant. If your pregnancy is high-risk, or if you have certain pre-existing medical conditions, some dental treatment may need to be postponed.

Although digital x-rays are considered safe during any stage of pregnancy (when abdominal and thyroid shielding is used), we try to minimize any exposure unless absolutely necessary.

Elective dental treatment should wait until after delivery. Elective treatment is anything that you don't need immediately and that is not necessary for your health or the health of your baby. However, if you need a filling, root canal or extraction, it is best to have it treated to prevent possible infection or complications. Treatment during any stage of pregnancy is safe, but the second trimester is the safest.

Many local anaesthetics (with or without epinephrine) are considered safe to use during pregnancy, however the benefits and risks to both the mother and fetus must still always be considered (J Dental Anesth Pain Med, 13). Nitrous oxide (laughing gas) should be avoided during pregnancy.

While it is best to avoid taking any medication during pregnancy, if an infection occurs antibiotics may be necessary, as well as pain medication. Before a drug can be labelled safe to take during pregnancy, it must undergo vigorous testing and research. Although no medicine is risk-free, antibiotics such as penicillin, amoxicillin and cephalosporins such as cephalexin have a long history of effectiveness and have shown themselves to be safe to use during all stages of pregnancy (Medicines in Pregnancy, 14). Tetracycline is avoided as it can cause tooth staining in the fetus (Mother to Baby, 15).

The FDA list of Pharmaceutical Pregnancy Categories outlines the prenatal safety of over-the-counter medications. There are five categories - A,B,C, D and X. Drugs in Category A and B have been found to be safe for use during pregnancy, whereas drugs in Category X should not be used by pregnant women (FDA Pregnancy Categories, 16). It is mandatory for all drugs to have the pregnancy category designation on its package insert. For pain management, over-the-counter acetaminophen (Tylenol) is listed in Category B and considered safe to use during pregnancy. NSAIDs (such as Advil) are not recommended during pregnancy, especially after week 20 (Mother to Baby, 17). Before taking any medication, always check with your prenatal provider first.

Lastly, oral hygiene habits may change due to morning sickness, a strong gag reflex or simple exhaustion. Patients can try using a smaller toothbrush to make brushing easier. Studies show that associations exist between pregnancy periodontitis and preterm delivery, low birth weight, gestational diabetes and development of preeclampsia. Although a causal relationship is yet to be confirmed, it is safe to maintain that good oral hygiene during pregnancy can help you have a healthy pregnancy and a healthy baby.

Medications

This chapter is essentially a "cheat sheet" of the most common medications that are prescribed in dentistry and what they are used to treat. It is only a reference and should not supersede the advice of your dentist. I won't go into too much detail on narcotics because I do not prescribe them often for reasons that are beyond this book. Narcotics are reserved for severe pain and even with all the work I do, I rarely encounter severe pain that cannot be controlled with over the counter Advil and Tylenol. I would say that 95% of post-operative pain management for my patients is a combination of Advil and Tylenol at therapeutic levels. What this means is that one Advil 200 mg is subtherapeutic and won't do much. Most tooth pain is inflammatory-based so NSAIDs (non-steroidal anti-inflammatory drugs) like Advil are your best friend. Most of the time, this is all you will need.

Painkillers

Let's begin with painkillers. There are different types of drugs for pain and each has different effects. Always use the lowest possible dose for the shortest possible time to relieve your symptoms. If your symptoms persist for more than 3 days, go see your dentist.

1. Advil/Ibuprofen/Motrin

    These are all the same, just under different names. For pain, 600 mg every 6 hours is recommended. You can use 800 mg as your first dose (to speed things up) but then stick to 600 mg thereafter. 200-400 mg is for pain and 400-600 mg is for the anti-inflammatory effect. This is the go-to regiment for any tooth pain. You can combine this with Tylenol to act in synergy but always start with ibuprofen first unless it's medically contraindicated. The maximum daily dose for an adult is 2400 mg.

    Contraindications include but are not limited to renal (kidney) impairment, GI issues (IBD/IBS), history of ulcers, bleeding issues and allergies. Always check with both your doctor and pharmacist.

Dosing for children is based on weight. The general recommendation is 5-10 mg/kg every 6 hours with a daily maximum of 40mg/kg/day. For example, if your child is 35 lbs (or 15.9 kg, rounding up to 16 kg) that would equal 80-160 mg every 6 hours, not to exceed 640mg daily. As long as you stick to the recommended dosage, you will be at or below the daily maximum but never over.

If your child is of average weight for their age, you can use this simplified version.

Age	Liquid form (160mg/5mL) 5mL is 1 Teaspoon	Chewable tablets (80mg)
4-11 months	½ Teaspoon	Not applicable
12-23 months	¾ Teaspoon	Not applicable
2-3 years	1 Teaspoon	2 tablets
4-5 years	1.5 Teaspoon	3 tablets
6-8 years	2 Teaspoons	4 tablets
9-10 years	2.5 Teaspoons	5 tablets
11-12 years	3 Teaspoons	6 tablets

2. Aleve/Naproxen

   This is another NSAID that works well for pain. Use 500 mg as a loading dose and then 250mg every 6 hours thereafter. The daily maximum is 1250 mg.

3. Tylenol/Acetaminophen

   Again, same drug, different names. For pain, 650mg every 6 hours is recommended. The maximum daily dose is 4000 mg.

   Tylenol is not an NSAID – it does not help reduce swelling or inflammation. It works mostly in the brain by blocking the release of substances that cause the feeling of pain. It is metabolized in the liver and contraindicated in those with liver issues as well as alcoholics. Avoid alcohol when taking Tylenol.

Dosing for children is again based on weight. The recommendation is 10-15 mg/kg every 4-6 hours with a maximum daily dose of 65mg/kg/day. Using the same 35 lb child (or 15.9 kg, rounded up to 16 kg), this would mean 160–240 mg every 4-6 hours, not to exceed 1040mg daily.

If your child is of average weight for their age, you can use this simplified version.

Age	Liquid form (160mg/5mL) 5mL is 1 Teaspoon	Chewable tablets (80mg)
4-11 months	½ Teaspoon	Not applicable
12-23 months	¾ Teaspoon	Not applicable
2-3 years	1 Teaspoon	2 tablets
4-5 years	1.5 Teaspoon	3 tablets
6-8 years	2 Teaspoons	4 tablets
9-10 years	2.5 Teaspoons	5 tablets
11-12 years	3 Teaspoons	6 tablets

Tylenol 3 is sometimes prescribed after the extraction of wisdom teeth. The recommendation is to take 1-2 tablets every 4-6 hours for pain. Tylenol 3 is a combination of 325 mg of acetaminophen, 30 mg of codeine and 15 mg of caffeine. Codeine is a narcotic drug that gets partially metabolized into morphine in the body. It should not be used by anyone with severe asthma or breathing problems, an allergy to acetaminophen or codeine, during pregnancy or while breastfeeding. If you are an ultra-rapid metabolizer, Tylenol 3 should not be used. Avoid driving or operating machinery as it can cause dizziness and drowsiness. Never drink alcohol while taking Tylenol 3.

Antibiotics

Let's move on to antibiotics. Antibiotics are prescribed to treat an infection or to prevent one. They work by killing bacteria or stopping them from spreading. When an oral infection occurs, the overgrowth of bacteria causes a pocket of pus to form. This often causes swelling and pain. If left untreated, the infection can spread to other areas of the jaw or even the brain. There are many different classes of antibiotics and within each class, individual antibiotics treat different types of infections.

1. Amoxicillin

    This is the go-to antibiotic for oral infections. It is widely effective and has the fewest gastrointestinal side effects. Take 500mg every 8 hours for 7 days. Your first dose can be doubled (1g) to speed things up. Amoxicillin is contraindicated if you are allergic to penicillin.

    For children, amoxicillin is normally given in liquid form and is based on age, weight and the type of infection being treated. The recommended range is 20-40mg/kg/day, in divided doses every 8 hours for 10 days (not to exceed 2g per day). For a child weighing 20kg, this would mean 400-800mg/day, or 133-267mg per dose. Assuming a suspension of 250mg/5mL and to make it easier to dispense, this translates to 1 teaspoon (5mL) every 8 hours.

2. Azithromycin

    Azithromycin is the second option if you are allergic to Amoxicillin. The standard is a loading dose of 500mg (day 1), followed by 250mg once a day for the next 4 days. Contraindications would include an allergy to azithromycin or other macrolide antibiotics.

    For children, dosing is based on weight and is provided in liquid form. The standard dosing recommendation is 5-12mg/kg taken as a single dose daily for 3 days. For a child weighing 20kg, this would mean 100-240mg daily. Assuming a suspension of 200mg/5mL and to make it easier to dispense, this translates to 1 teaspoon (5mL) daily.

For any antibiotic, always make sure that you take the full course prescribed, even if you start to feel better before finishing them. If the full course is not completed, you may not kill off the bacteria, which can lead to recurring infections and antibiotic resistance.

Antibiotic premedication (taken from RCDSO, 18 and AHA, 19)

In dentistry, antibiotic premedication or antibiotic prophylaxis refers to the taking of antibiotics before certain dental procedures (ones that may cause bleeding) to decrease the chance of infection in another part of your body. For most people, this is not a concern but in persons at "high risk" of infection or with certain heart conditions, it is absolutely necessary. We no longer provide antibiotic coverage for any joint replacement, however your orthopaedic surgeon may still want you on premedication and that is up to their discretion.

Antibiotic coverage is still required for patients who have cardiac conditions that put them at greatest risk for adverse outcomes from infective endocarditis (an infection of the heart's inner lining or heart valves). These include patients who have:

1. A prosthetic cardiac valve
2. A prosthetic cardiac valve repair
3. A history of infective endocarditis
4. Specific congenital (present from birth) heart disease (CHD) including:
    a. Unrepaired cyanotic CHD including palliative shunts and conduits
    b. Completely repaired CHD with prosthetic material or device – whether placed by surgery or catheter intervention, during the first 6 months after procedure
    c. Repaired CHD with residual defects at the site or adjacent to the site of a prosthetic patch or a prosthetic device (which inhibit endothelialisation)

5. Cardiac transplantation recipients who develop cardiac valvulopathy

The standard is a single dose of 2g of Amoxicillin (or four 500mg capsules) 30-60 minutes before your appointment.

For those who are allergic to penicillin, the standard a single dose of 500mg of Azithromycin 30-60 minutes before your procedure.

For patients who need repeated dental procedures that might introduce bacteria into the bloodstream, the recommendation is to use an antibiotic from a different class or to wait at least 4 weeks between treatment sessions.

For those patients who might already be on a short course (7–10 days) of oral antibiotics, it is recommended that an antibiotic from a different class be used for prophylaxis coverage or to delay the dental procedure for at least 10 days after completion of the short course of antibiotic.

Other common medications

There are some other medications commonly used or prescribed in dentistry. I have listed them below.

1. Decadron/Dexamethasone

    This is a steroid used to decrease swelling and inflammation after surgery. It is mainly prescribed as a single dose (4mg) pre-surgery. If it is a more extensive surgery involving a patient with a complicated medical history, there will be multiple doses. The exact protocol will be determined by your doctor. Dexamethasone is also used for post-operative paraesthesia or nerve issues.

2. Chlorohexidine (CHX)

    This is a common mouth rinse prescribed for use after surgery. It can cause severe staining if used for longer than 2 weeks. Recent research has made this rinse less popular, when compared with the use of CPC (below).

3. Crest Pro Health (Cetylpyridinium Chloride CPC)

   This is an over-the-counter mouth rinse. It can also cause staining with long term use.

4. Triazolam

   This is the main sedative used in oral moderate sedation. It is a benzodiazepine and is usually given as a 0.25mg – 0.50mg dose one hour prior to surgery, in the dental office. It works quickly and does not stay in your system long due to its short half-life. Sometimes other less potent benzodiazepines are given prior to surgery as an anti-anxiety like Ativan (lorazepam) or Valium (diazepam). These will last longer in your system but aren't as strong.

Remember to follow the instructions given by your doctor and pharmacist when it comes to any medication. Always provide your entire medical history regardless of how important you believe it to be. If you get an allergic reaction (most commonly hives, rash and itching) to any medication, stop it right away and call your doctor. Make sure you review the common side effects of any medication with your pharmacist so you know what is normal and what is not.

Post-op Instructions

I have included some post-op instructions for various procedures so you always have something to reference. Keep in mind that these may change depending on your doctor, however the principles remain the same. Always follow their instructions.

Oral Surgery

It is not unusual for swelling to occur after surgery. Swelling often peaks 2-3 days after the procedure and may take 4-7 days to subside.

- Apply an ice pack to the outside of your face - 20 minutes on/off for 6-8 hours after the surgery. This will help keep the swelling to a minimum but may not completely eliminate it. It is not uncommon for swelling to occur until the day following surgery.

A small amount of bleeding can be expected for the first few hours after the surgery.

- If there is considerable bleeding, apply pressure to the area by biting down on a rolled piece of gauze for 20 minutes until the bleeding stops. Do not remove the gauze during this period to examine the surgical site. If bleeding persists, call the office. Do not try to stop the bleeding by rinsing or spitting. This will cause the area to bleed more. It is recommended that you place a towel over your pillow the first night after surgery.

A certain amount of discomfort can be expected following surgery.

- Take painkillers as directed. Avoid taking it on an empty stomach to prevent nausea.

Do not drink through a straw for 24 hours after surgery. Avoid rinsing during this time also.

- Sucking and swishing motions can dislodge the blood clots which can lead to dry sockets, increased pain and delayed healing.

Post-op Instructions

A proper diet is essential to healing. Chew on the non-operated side of your mouth, if possible.

- Soft foods such as mashed potatoes, soups, apple sauce and shakes are recommended for the first post-operative days.
- Stay away from sharp little foods such as popcorn, potato chips, etc.
- Avoid citrus juices, highly spiced foods and alcohol – they will cause pain.

Do not smoke for at least 7 days after surgery. Heat and smoke can break down the blood clot,

cause dry socket, increase pain and delay healing. It can also irritate your gums.

You may experience a slight feeling of weakness and chills during the first 24 hours.

- Follow your regular daily activities but avoid excessive exertion of any type. Activities such as going to the gym, golfing, tennis, skiing, swimming etc. should be postponed for a few days after surgery. Quiet activity is recommended for the first 48 hours after surgery.

A follow up 7-10 days later may be required to ensure proper healing regardless of how the surgery area looks or feels.

Implants

Implant post-op instructions are the same as oral surgery post-op instructions, with the following special considerations.

- With ceramic implants, make sure to wear your Essix retainer 24 HOURS PER DAY for 3 months until it is ready to restore. Only remove AFTER eating to rinse it out and clean it. Eat with it. Sleep with it.
- Avoid touching the implant area with your fingers, tongue or toothbrush unless otherwise directed by your doctor.

- You can use a Monoject syringe with salt water rinse or Crest Pro Health (Cetylpyridinium Chloride CPC). Your doctor will provide a post-surgical soft brush to clean that area after the stitches are removed.

With any oral surgical procedure, LESS IS MORE. The less you do to the surgical site, the better it will heal.

Sedation (with Triazolam)

The sedative will take time to clear your system. This can take anywhere from 12-24 hours. It is important that you rest and be carefully monitored for 24 hours after your appointment.

There should be no outside activity for the remainder of the day following the procedure. After that time, activity may be resumed based on the surgery and other post-treatment considerations. You should remain in a reclined position for the rest of the day, except to go the bathroom. Someone must accompany/support you when walking.

For the first 24 hours after sedation :

- Do not drive.
- Do not operate machinery or potentially dangerous equipment.
- Do not make any important decisions or sign any important documents.
- Do not consume any alcoholic beverages.
- Do not engage in any activities that require coordination.

You should be able to eat and drink normally, subject to restrictions placed by the type of dental procedure that was done. Eating is only dictated by the way you feel. Drink lots of fluid.

Nausea is a possible side effect of sedation. Pain medication and/or antibiotics on an empty stomach can also cause of nausea. It is best to take these types of medication with food to prevent nausea. If nausea persists for longer than 4 hours, contact your dental office so appropriate management can be instituted.

Post-operatively, do not take any narcotic pain medication (codeine, Percodan® and others) until 8 hours after you take the Triazolam. **Soft Tissue Graft**

Relax for the remainder of the day. It is best to refrain from strenuous physical activity, heavy lifting or bending over for the next few days. This will help reduce pain, swelling and prevent additional bleeding.

For the first 2 weeks after surgery, do not smoke or consume alcohol. Both of these will delay the healing process and can increase the incidence of complications.

Swelling is normal after the surgery and can peak 2-5 days after surgery.

- Apply an ice pack to the outside of your face - 20 minutes on/off for the first 24 hours. This will help keep the swelling to a minimum but may not completely eliminate it.

Most of the bleeding will have stopped once you leave the office.

- It is normal for your saliva to be a reddish colour for the first 24 hours.
- If excessive bleeding occurs, place a moist gauze on the surgical area and hold firmly but gently for 20 minutes. Do not put the gauze on dry otherwise it can stick to the stitches and pull everything out.
- Avoid any negative or positive pressure which can dislodge the clot. Avoid drinking through a straw, forceful spitting, rinsing with your mouth closed or blowing your nose forcefully.

A certain amount of discomfort can be expected following surgery.

- Discomfort can last anywhere from a few days to the first few weeks. Most patients are pain-free after 3 days.
- Take medications as recommended by your Doctor. Avoid taking painkillers on an empty stomach to prevent nausea.

Stitches are placed to hold the gums in the proper position during healing.

- Avoid looking at the graft site. Minimize movement of the lips and do not pull on your lips to look at the graft - these actions can increase bleeding and cause the stitches to come undone.
- Do not disturb the sutures with your tongue or toothbrush.
- Stitches are normally removed 2 weeks after the surgery. If a stitch starts to come loose, do not pull it out. Wait for it to come out on its own or until your follow up.

During the course of healing, the tissue graft may change appearance and color. The color may appear white/gray/red during the healing period. This is normal. Do NOT be alarmed by the appearance of the graft.

A proper diet is essential to healing. Chew away from the surgical site for the first 2 weeks until the stitches are removed.

- Soft foods are recommended. This means anything that does not need to be cut or that can be cut with a fork - mashed potatoes, soups, eggs, fish, apple sauce, shakes, etc.
- Stay away from sharp little foods (no popcorn, potato chips etc.).
- Avoid hot, spicy or acidic foods and drinks for the first few days.

Maintain a normal level of oral hygiene.

- Continue to brush and floss the teeth which were NOT involved in the surgery.
- Do not brush, floss or touch the surgical area for 10 days after the surgery.
- You can use a salt water rinse or Crest Pro Health (Cetylpyridinium Chloride CPC) the day AFTER surgery. Do not use any other mouthwashes.

Post-op Instructions

- You will be given a special toothbrush to use in the surgical area at your follow-up appointment.

Nightguards

It may take a while to get used to wearing your nightguard. Always place your nightguard in hot water for 5-10 seconds to soften it before wearing – this will make it easier to fit in your mouth.

- If you notice that the nightguard feels too tight anywhere (shifting/pushing of any of your teeth), please let us know so we can adjust it.
- The bite may also need to be adjusted to make it more comfortable.

When you remove your nightguard in the morning, always clean it. No matter what you use, nightguards will discolour and get cloudy over time. This is normal.

- Use a soft-bristled toothbrush with a bit of toothpaste (nothing too abrasive). Rinse well after.
- Avoid using anything with alcohol (check your mouthwash label) as this can crack the acrylic over time.
- Allow to air dry completely before storing in any closed container.
- Never place your nightguard in the dishwasher or boil in water to clean.

Bring your nightguard in with you for any dental visit. We can clean it and make any necessary adjustments.

- Always bring your nightguard if you are having any restorative treatment (fillings, crowns, etc.)

Dogs love nightguards. They make great chew toys. Please store them safety, out of reach of furry friends.

Invisalign

The success of any Invisalign treatment is dependent on patient compliance. Aligners should be worn at least 22 hours a day. They should only be removed for eating, drinking anything other than water and brushing.

- Always brush and floss after eating before placing trays back in otherwise you will get cavities.
- Do not brush immediately after having anything acidic. Wait 30 minutes before brushing and reinserting your aligner.
- When brushing your teeth, brush off your aligners as well.
- Always brush your teeth and aligners in the morning.
- Never place aligners in boiling water or soak them in mouthwash or denture cleaner.

The first tray and the first day of most trays will feel tight as they are moving your teeth to the next stage. This is normal.

- When inserting your aligners, always place them front to back. Begin with your front teeth and gently move backward.
- When removing your aligners, remove from back to front. Begin with your back teeth and gently wiggle your way forward. Do not remove aligners by pulling straight down from the back. This can crack the aligner in the middle.
- Change your trays according to the schedule provided by your Doctor (usually 1 week changes). Change them at night just before you go to bed so you can get used to the new trays while you sleep.
- The trays are made to be worn sequentially so don't skip trays.
- If the next set of trays don't fit, try wearing your last tray for an extra day to see if that helps – if not please call the office.

Post-op Instructions

- Use Chewies to help seat your trays every time you take them out – this will help them track.

- Your teeth are shifting so your bite will be changing and teeth may start to feel a little bit mobile. You may also have pain on a few trays. These usually go away. If they do not, please let your Doctor know.

Never place or wrap your aligners in a napkin - they can mistakenly get thrown away. Always store your trays in the Invisalign carrying case provided.

Keep your aligners away from pets. Dogs and cats think they are great chew toys.

If any attachments fall off, please call the office right away so we can place them back on, otherwise the next set of trays may not fit.

Never discard your aligners.

- When you are finished with a set, clean them and place them back in their original pouch. These can be used as back-ups in case an aligner is lost or broken.

- If you misplace or break a set of aligners, wear the previous set. Call the office to discuss next steps.

It is important that your progress be monitored.

- Keep all appointments.

- If doing virtual care progress, remember to upload your photos at your designated intervals.

Upon completion of your Invisalign treatment, you will need to wear retainers to prevent relapse. Remember, there is nothing we do in your mouth that you cannot undo.

References

1. Kois Learning Center - https://www.koiscenter.com/patient-education/miscellaneous/how-much-radiation-do-i-get-from-a-dental-x-ray

2. ADA – Patient Smart – Baby Bottle Tooth Decay - https://www.ada.org/~/media/ADA/Publications/Files/ADA_Patient_Smart_BBTD.ashx

3. ADA – MouthHealthy - https://www.mouthhealthy.org/en/az-topics/e/eruption-charts

4. Huff Post – Parent to Parent: All you need to know about your childrens teeth - https://www.huffpost.com/entry/parent-to-parent-all-you-_b_9825940

5. ADA – Fluoridation facts - https://www.ada.org/~/media/ADA/Files/Fluoridation_Facts.pdf?la=en

6. "The Effect of Toothbrushing and Flossing Sequence on Interdental Plaque Reduction and Fluoride Retention: A Randomized Controlled Clinical Trial", Journal of Periodontology 2018 - https://aap.onlinelibrary.wiley.com/doi/abs/10.1002/JPER.17-0149

7. Dental Care – https://www.dentalcare.com/en-us/professional-education/ce-courses/ce542/tooth-whitening

8. Science Direct – Agreement among dentists' restorative treatment planning thresholds for primary occlusal caries, primary proximal caries, and existing restorations: Findings from the national dental practice-based research network- https://www.sciencedirect.com/science/article/abs/pii/S0300571213001371

9. Tooth whitening – *what we need to know by Clifton M Carey* - https://www.ncbi.nlm.nih.gov/pmc/articles/PMC4058574

10. Glidewell Overdenture- https://glidewelldental.com/solutions/implant-solutions/implant-restorations/implant-overdentures

References

11. Glidewell All on X - https://glidewelldental.com/solutions/implant-solutions/implant-restorations/bruxzir-esthetic-implant-prosthesis

12. Dental Care – https://www.dentalcare.com/en-us/professional-education/ce-courses/ce542/tooth-whitening

13. Journal of Dent Anesthesia and Pain Medicine - Use of local Anesthetics for dental treatment during pregnancy https://www.ncbi.nlm.nih.gov/pmc/articles/PMC5564152/

14. Medicines in Pregnancy - https://www.medicinesinpregnancy.org/Medicine--pregnancy/Amoxicillin/

15. Mother to Baby - https://mothertobaby.org/fact-sheets/tetracycline-pregnancy/

16. FDA Pregnancy Categories - https://www.drugs.com/pregnancy-categories.html

17. Mother to Baby - https://mothertobaby.org/fact-sheets/ibuprofen-pregnancy/pdf

18. RCDSO Prophylaxis Recommendations - https://www.rcdso.org/en-ca/rcdso-members/practice-advisory-service/information-on-antibiotic-prophylaxis

19. ADA Scientific Statement - Prevention of Viridans Group Streptococcal Infective Endocarditis - https://www.ahajournals.org/doi/pdf/10.1161/CIR.0000000000000969

www.ingramcontent.com/pod-product-compliance
Lightning Source LLC
Chambersburg PA
CBHW070436220526
45466CB00004B/1698